HORMONES

the woman's answer book

HORMONES

L. Jovanovic and G. S. Sharpe

Edited and adapted by
Peter D. O'Neill, B.A. (Hons), M.Phil.

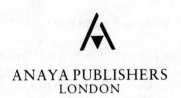

ANAYA PUBLISHERS
LONDON

*This book is dedicated to our mothers
and to women who may, at times,
feel they are ruled by inner forces
they do not understand*

First published in Great Britain 1990
by Anaya Publishers Ltd, 49 Neal St, London WC2H 9PJ
Originally published in the United States of America in 1987 by
Atheneum Publishers Inc., a division of Macmillan Publishing Company,
866 Third Avenue, New York, N.Y. 10022

British Library Cataloguing in Publication Data
A CIP catalogue record for this book is available from the British Library
ISBN 1–85470–020–0
Typeset by Keyspools Ltd, Golborne, Lancs
Printed in Great Britain by
Redwood Press Limited, Melksham, Wiltshire

The illustration on page 109 is adapted from information in J. Ginsburg
et al., 'Cardiovascular responses during the hot flush', *Br. J. Obstet.
Gynaecol*, 1981, 88, pp 925–30, and appears by kind permission of the
publishers and authors.

Special Adviser for the Anaya edition:

Jean Ginsburg, MA, DM, FRCP

Consultant Endocrinologist, Royal Free Hospital
and Senior Lecturer in Endocrinology,
Royal Free Hospital School of Medicine, London

Contents

CONTENTS

CONTENTS

INTRODUCTION

Most of us give very little thought to how our bodies work until something goes wrong. We are generally aware of the fact that our glands produce hormones, but many people, including too many doctors, lack a clear understanding of just how important hormones are.

Women need to learn about the way that hormones influence not only their physical wellbeing, but also their mental lives. A well-informed patient is better able to participate intelligently in important health choices and decisions. Prevention succeeds by spotting early warning signs; knowing that a troublesome symptom is simply a variation of what is normal and shared by millions, is also reassuring. Fear is said to be a lack of knowledge. *Hormone therapy must be conducted under expert care. You should ensure that you consult with your doctor or other medical experts before undertaking any course of treatment to be sure that you need it and if it is the correct one.*

There are socio-political reasons why women should learn more about their bodies. A woman experiences cyclical changes in her body and she has the ability to bear children. These factors have been, and are still, used by some in positions of management and authority (mainly men but some women too, unfortunately) to discriminate against women. The PMT (pre-menstrual tension) debate may have polarised positions further between those who try to claim women are 'unreliable' because of hormone surges, and campaigning women. The latter are better able now to show that the medical profession in the past has been poorly informed about the complexities of women's hormonal systems and produced, not only wrong, but damaging diagnoses of what is a normal situation.

The fact is, hormones govern almost every facet of the body's activities for both males and females of all ages. By understanding the roles of these vital substances we can take the steps needed to lead more harmonious and satisfying lives.

The aim of this book is to clear up many common misconceptions. It does not shy away from the technical. Hormonal systems are complex and effort is needed to understand them. But, by giving detailed information, it should help women to make informed health decisions on many topics, from treating acne and dieting, to deciding on a method of contraception and whether to consider taking oestrogen supplements following menopause. Doctors are trained to use technical terms but rarely to communicate what they mean, so there is an extensive glossary at the back of the book with an explanation of many of the terms. Here is a brief resume of some major areas.

Glands

A gland is an organ or structure which produces secretions. Obvious ones are the sweat and salivary glands. These are *exocrine* glands, which have ducts to carry their secretions externally. This book looks mainly at *endocrine* glands, a finely tuned network of ductless glands which secrete dozens of different chemical compounds, called hormones, directly into the bloodstream. These include glands such as the thyroid, pituitary, pineal, parathyroid, thymus, adrenal, pancreas, and the gonads (the ovaries in women and the testes in men). A number of organs also secrete important hormones, including the brain, kidneys, lungs, heart and intestinal lining.

Hormones

Hormones are chemical messengers which control scores of vital processes and act on virtually every cell of the body. The glands which produce them work with each other and the nervous system, through a finely tuned feedback network, and release specific hormones which carry messages to other parts of the body and to trigger specific responses.

For example, when a baby begins to breastfeed, its sucking sends a message, in a millisecond, along the mother's nerves and spinal cord to the hypothalamus area of her brain. The message signals the hypothalamus to tell the pituitary to release a hormone called oxytocin into the blood. In a few seconds, the oxytocin reaches the milk ducts in the breast, causing them to contract and release a flow of milk. During the process, the pituitary releases another hormone, prolactin, which plays a key role in the production of breastmilk. Sometimes, just the sound of a crying, hungry baby provides enough stimulation to cause the message to be sent to the mother's brain. This oversimplified explanation gives a basic idea of the general process.

Hormones influence growth, sexual development and desire, our metabolism, muscular development, mental acuity, behaviour and our sleep cycles. They enable us to respond quickly to a dangerous situation by putting the body on full alert and help to maintain the proper internal, chemical and fluid balances.

Some hormones act directly on an organ to produce a desired effect, as with breastfeeding. Some hormones simply have the job of triggering other endocrine glands to go into action. They are called *trophic* hormones and include those which stimulate the thyroid to secrete its hormones, and the gonadotrophins which stimulate the ovaries and testes to produce their respective hormones.

Endocrinology
This is the branch of science and medicine devoted to the endocrine system. An endocrinologist specialises in disorders of the endocrine system. Some specialise further in different areas such as reproduction, or paediatric endocrinology which deals with growth and development in children.

Despite its complexity the endocrine system is very stable and disorders are rare. Often, what may appear to be a glandular problem is in fact caused by something else. An overweight person may rationalise that they are fat because of a thyroid problem, when it is their diet that is at fault. But this book is as much about understanding how to time and respond to our hormonal systems, as recognising that things may be going wrong. It is important to understand how normal hormonal functions affect us. The fluctuations of the monthly cycle can cause mood changes and PMT. Knowing what is going on is an essential factor in ensuring they do not upset your equilibrium. Young girls should not find themselves upset and alarmed at changes in their bodies simply because they are deprived of information.

Oestrogen replacement therapy may have an important role to play for some women in tackling the problems caused by a thinning of the bones (osteoporosis). But decisions about this should be based on an understanding of the role of calcium metabolism and menopause. In Part I of the book the various endocrine glands and hormones are described in detail. Part II is devoted to the roles hormones play in the stages of a woman's life, from childhood to old age. Part III describes a variety of hormone-related disorders and how they may be treated.

PART I

Hormones: How They Rule Your Life

CHAPTER ONE

The Endocrine System – An Overview

CHILDREN ask scores of difficult, if not 'unanswerable', questions about what makes us different from each other. Why is Daddy different from Mummy? Why are some people tall and others short? What makes me fall asleep at night and wakes me up in the morning? Why does Jimmy get angry so often? Why is Johnny's voice getting deeper? Why does Mummy have breasts and when will I grow mine?

The answers can be found in studying the endocrine system. Working in close cooperation with the nervous system, it keeps us 'in tune' with ourselves and our environment. It also produces the hormones that help make us unique.

To a large extent, hormones determine whether we will be tall or short, fat or thin, calm or nervous, fast-moving or slow. The endocrine system enables us to adapt to a constantly changing environment, to cope with the stresses of daily life and to reproduce and fulfil our biological functions as human beings. Many of these processes take place without any conscious thought or action. Both the endocrine and our nervous systems have messengers that are responsible for thousands of different automatic responses and, together, they regulate and integrate bodily functions.

The nervous system is like a telephone. Messages are carried by electrical impulses along a network of specialised cells, called neurons, to a specific receptor, the 'person' receiving your call. Neural responses are virtually instantaneous – if you touch a hot stove, the sensory nerves in your fingers send out a pain message and your hand is automatically jerked away before you even have time to think about it.

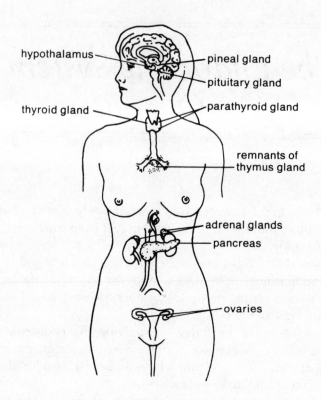

hypothalamus —
pineal gland
pituitary gland
thyroid gland —
parathyroid gland
remnants of thymus gland
adrenal glands
pancreas
ovaries

Figure 1. The female endocrine system

In contrast, in the endocrine system the messengers are chemical and either reside locally or travel via the bloodstream to receptors. The latter are specialised cells in the various organs or body tissues that are specially programmed to receive them, or to tell them to go on somewhere else in the body. These chemical messengers are, of course, hormones. They are produced by endocrine glands, the hypothalamus area of the brain, and tissues scattered throughout the body. Working through an elaborate, exceedingly sensitive and fine-tuned communications system, the various glands secrete hormones as needed to regulate bodily functions. Since hormones, in effect, travel by water instead of the electrical impulses used by the nervous system, their responses are somewhat slower than neural reactions.

The endocrine glands

The major endocrine glands are pictured in Figure 1. Hormones are also manufactured in glandular tissue located in organs such as the intestines, lungs and heart.

Every now and then, researchers discover unidentified hormones, and new things are constantly being learned about known ones.

To give a clearer picture of just how important the endocrine system and its hormones are, here is a brief description of the major glands, their hormones and their myriad functions.

The pituitary

Located deep inside the head, the pituitary lies behind the nasal cavities and just below the hypothalamus. The hypothalamus is part of the forebrain, or diencephalon. This is often referred to as the 'old', or original, brain and is the seat of primitive instincts – hunger, thirst, sleep, procreation, self-defence – needed for the survival of the species. As humans evolved, new areas of the brain developed, specifically the cerebral cortex, which is the seat of intelligence. The hypothalamus links this thinking part of the brain and the pituitary gland. Both the hypothalamus and the pituitary produce many of the hormones that control other glands. But it is the hypothalamus that is the first 'controller', sending signals to the pituitary to activate it and in turn make it send out hormones. The pituitary is divided into a lobe at the front (anterior lobe) and a lobe at the back (posterior), an extension of the hypothalamus, nerve-like in its makeup.

Hormones produced in the pituitary's anterior lobe are mostly trophic hormones, meaning that they stimulate other glands or organs to go into action. For example, hormones known as gonado-trophins are produced here. In a woman, these include follicle-stimulating hormone (FSH), which prompts the ovaries to ripen an egg each month, and luteinizing hormone (LH), which stimulates the ovarian follicle to release the ripened egg. In males, FSH stimulates sperm production and LH, male hormone (testosterone) production. LH is also involved in sperm maturation.

Other anterior pituitary hormones include: growth-stimulating hormone, or somatotrophin, which is responsible for a child's growth; adreno-corticotrophic hormone (ACTH), which acts to stimulate the adrenal glands to produce their hormones; thyroid-

17

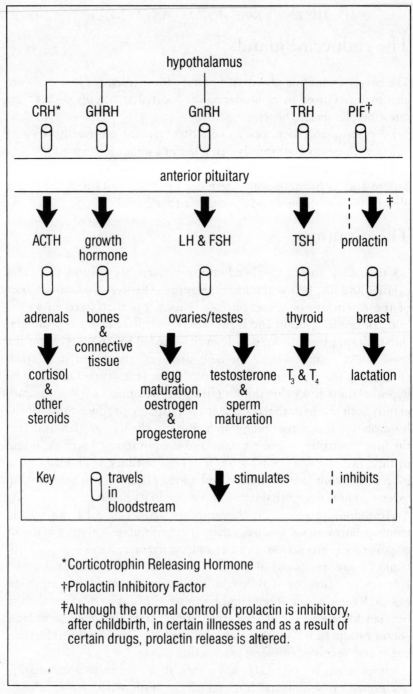

Figure 2. How the hypothalamus and pituitary relate to other endocrine glands

stimulating hormone (TSH), which stimulates the thyroid gland to produce its hormones; and prolactin, which stimulates the breasts to produce milk.

Two hormones are secreted from the pituitary's posterior lobe: vasopressin is an anti-diuretic hormone that helps the kidneys conserve water and maintain the body's fluid balance. It may also be involved in the tone of blood vessels. An absence of vasopressin results in diabetes insipidus, a condition marked by excessive thirst and over-production of urine. The other hormone, oxytocin, promotes uterine contractions during labour and also stimulates the breasts to give up their milk.

The hypothalamus regulates and coordinates many endocrine functions, especially through its control of the pituitary gland, (see Figure 2). It produces stimulating, trophic hormones which reach the pituitary through a special network of blood vessels. Expert views vary but symptoms or disorders with psychological or emotional roots may involve the relationship between the hypothalamus and the pituitary. Our appetite control centre is thought to be in the hypothalamus and the cause of some eating disorders, such as anorexia nervosa or bulimia, may stem from a disturbance in that region and in turn be influenced by higher centres in the brain.

Severe emotional distress or weight loss because of illness and so forth, may act on higher centres of the brain but also affect the hypothalamus. Periods may stop partly through a lack of hormones produced by the hypothalamus.

Too much growth hormone can result in giantism and a lack of gonadotrophins in dwarfism. Too early a release of the sex hormones (gonadotrophins) may cause premature sexual development, but if they are not released at puberty then the body will not mature sexually. Lack of gonadotrophins may also be a cause of infertility in women. Over-production of prolactin may cause abnormal production of breastmilk and failure to menstruate. In the rare event of the anterior pituitary lobe being destroyed, the genitals shrink, there is impotence in men and infertility in women, low blood pressure, slowed heart rate and lethargy. We have difficulty fighting off infection, tolerate the cold poorly, age prematurely and face increasing disability which leads to premature death. Pituitary function can fail due to haemorrhage after childbirth because the hormone-distributing network of blood vessels is damaged. It may also occur after trauma from a head injury in a road traffic accident. But hormone replacement can help in preventing or minimising many of these effects.

The thyroid

Moving down the body, the next major endocrine gland we encounter is the thyroid, a butterfly-shaped structure that lies over the windpipe and just below the larynx. Normally the thyroid weighs 25g (1oz) or less. Its hormones are essential to proper metabolism and a failure of the thyroid can affect virtually every organ and system in the body.

The thyroid secretes three hormones – triiodothyronine (T3) and thyroxine (T4), which control metabolism by increasing the oxygen consumption of cells, and calcitonin, which is involved in calcium metabolism. The T3 and T4 thyroid hormones are involved in the normal growth and development of the brain, muscles and bones, as well as the functioning of other endocrine glands and organ systems. A baby born with a thyroid deficiency is in danger of developing cretinism, a severe, irreversible form of mental retardation. Too much thyroid hormone increases the rate of metabolism causing, amongst other symptoms, a rapid heart beat. Too little results in a slowdown of almost all bodily processes. A goitre is the term used for swelling of the thyroid gland, either in whole or part and may be caused by too little (hypothyroidism) or too much thyroid hormone (hyperthyroidism). This is usually due to a lack of iodine but this is now relatively rare in industrialised countries. Hypothyroidism in menstruating women may cause heavier and more frequent periods because the ovaries fail to produce an egg each month.

The parathyroid

The parathyroid glands are small, disc-shaped structures which normally lie on the back and side of each thyroid lobe. Most of us have four of these tiny glands. The parathyroid hormone raises the amount of calcium circulating in the bloodstream while calcitonin (produced by the thyroid) lowers it.

Small amounts of calcium are needed for muscles and nerves to function properly; it is also essential for normal metabolism and clotting of the blood. By far the most plentiful mineral in the body, around 1kg (2.2lb) in the average adult, calcium is found mainly in

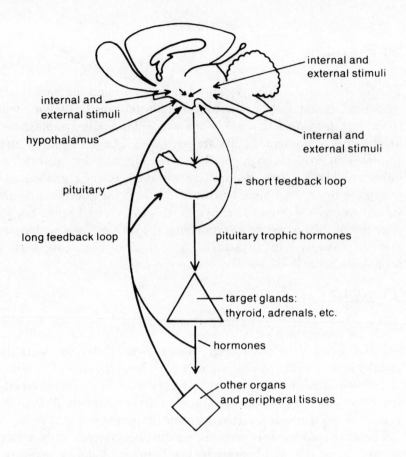

Figure 3. The hormone feedback system

the bones with small amounts circulating in the blood. When the level of the latter falls, parathyroid hormone is secreted to prompt the bones to release some of their store into the blood. Parathyroid hormone makes the kidneys increase the excretion of phosphate from the body and this increases the amount of calcium circulating in the blood. A lack of this hormone can cause severe muscle paralysis (tetany); if it affects the larynx, and it is not treated, a person may be suffocated.

The thyroid also produces calcitonin, whose exact function and action is unknown, but it is thought to influence calcium metabolism. Then again, removal of the thyroid does not change circulating calcium levels. Too much calcium in the blood may result in kidney stones, mental changes, irritability, high blood pressure and stomach ulcers.

The thymus

The function of the thymus gland, which lies behind the breastbone (sternum), is not fully understood. Made up mostly of lymphoid tissue, it is instrumental in producing white blood cells (lymphocytes) for the immune system. Babies are born with a large thymus, which continues to grow through childhood, reaching maturity just before puberty, when it starts gradually to shrink. It is quite small in old people or those who have had prolonged, severe infections or are subject to unusual stress. The thymus may be involved in the body's rejection of foreign tissue, but removing the thymus, as is sometimes done in patients with myasthenia gravis, does not cause such a profound change in the usual rejection response.

The adrenals

These are triangular-shaped and rest atop the kidneys; each is divided into two parts – the outer layer (cortex), which produces steroids, and the inner portion (medulla), which produces the stress hormones (catecholamines). Essentially, however, the medulla produces mainly adrenaline. Noradrenaline is produced at nerve terminals all over the body so is less dependent on the adrenals for production.

There are three types of steroids: (1) the mineralocorticoids, which control the body's fluid balance by regulating the kidneys' reabsorption of sodium and potassium; (2) the glucocorticoids, which help regulate the metabolism of blood sugar (glucose) and other nutrients, maintain blood pressure and enable the body to respond to physical stress; and (3) the sex hormones (androgens and oestrogens), which function similarly to those produced in the ovaries or testes.

The adrenal medulla's catecholamines include adrenaline (epinephrine) and noradrenaline (norepinephrine). Catecholamines are produced by other body tissues, so a person can get by without an adrenal medulla. The cortex and its hormones are vital to life and involved in intricate feedback systems that prompt the release of certain pituitary hormones.

Aldosterone is the major mineralocorticoid produced in the adrenal cortex. Its major role is to help the kidneys conserve sodium and thereby maintain the body's fluid balance. Its secretion is related to a feedback system involving ACTH (from the pituitary) in a minor way, and the blood levels of sodium, potassium and angiotensin II (which helps regulate blood pressure). Too much adlosterone leads to excessive sodium retention, high blood pressure and depletion of potassium. This can cause irregular heart beats, muscular weakness and cramps. Most instances of hyperaldosteronism can be traced to the growth of a tumour producing the hormone. Treatment is by removal of the tumour. If it is caused by an overactive gland, drugs may be prescribed.

Hydrocortisone is the most abundant of the glucocorticoids in humans; corticosterone, which has some mineralocorticoid function, is produced in lesser quantities. The liver can metabolise cortisol into hydrocortisone, a steroid that can also be manufactured and is given to patients with adrenal failure, or for some cases of severe allergic disorders.

The glucocorticoids affect metabolism in several ways. Hydrocortisone has an anti-insulin effect and is instrumental in transforming protein and fats into glucose – the body's major fuel. The adrenals increase hydrocortisone production following stress or injury. The instant danger is perceived, the brain sends a signal to the pituitary gland to produce ACTH, which, in turn, tells the adrenals to pump out extra hydrocortisone as well as catecholamines.

Cortisol production is also influenced by our internal biological clocks. Even in the absence of stress, the pituitary secretes spurts of ACTH throughout the 24-hour day. They are more frequent during the pre-dawn hours, accounting for our sleeping/waking patterns and perhaps part of the cause of jet lag when we travel across several time zones. However, the pineal gland is probably the main controlling factor in the latter.

Prolonged steroid therapy makes our own steroid-producing glands shrink and become sluggish. When the drugs are stopped abruptly the body cannot respond at speed to threats and it can suffer serious shock with all that entails. In Addison's disease (see Chapter 12) the adrenal glands are gradually destroyed and the body is exposed again to the dangers of poor responses to the so-called 'fight or flight' stresses. Cushing's syndrome (see Chapter 12) is related to over-production of glucocorticoids.

Sex hormones produced by the adrenals supplement those secreted by the ovaries and testes. The male sex hormones (androgens) produced by the adrenal glands in women influence the growth of their pubic and other body hair and their sex drives. Too much androgen production in a woman can prompt signs of masculinisation, and perhaps heightened sex drive.

The pancreas

This is a long, narrow organ extending across much of the upper abdomen. It is both an endocrine gland – with specialist cells that produce insulin and glucagon which are essential for metabolism and glucose balance – and an exocrine gland, producing digestive enzymes which travel through pancreatic ducts to the small intestine to aid in digestion.

Insulin, glucagon and somatostatin (the latter being a locally produced hormone as mentioned before) are manufactured in the Islets of Langerhans, collections of specialised cells scattered through the pancreas. Insulin, which is produced in the islets' beta cells, is crucial to the body's ability to break down carbohydrates and to utilise blood sugar (glucose). If not enough is produced then the body cannot cope with sugar it takes in or produces itself and diabetes results.

Glucagon, which is secreted by the islets' alpha cells, stimulates the liver to break down glycogen (stored blood sugar) and to return it to the bloodstream for use as fuel. When blood sugar falls, glucagon production rises, thus helping maintain a steady supply of glucose; it also enhances the conversion of protein to glucose. Somatostatin, which is produced in the islets' delta cells, inhibits alpha and beta cell production, so suppressing insulin and glucagon secretion and maintaining a balance.

The gonads

Sex hormones are greatly misunderstood. With the onset of puberty, hormones from the hypothalamus and pituitary set in motion changes in the activity of the reproductive organs – the testes in males and the ovaries in females. These ensure the increased development and operation of bodily changes which characterise puberty. Both men and women secrete each other's sex hormones; the difference, of course, lies in the relative balance – more oestrogen in women and more testosterone in men. Sexual development is discussed later in the book (see Index), but basically men get their 'maleness' from androgens, and women, their femininity from oestrogens. Male

testosterone (male hormone)   oestradiol (female hormone)

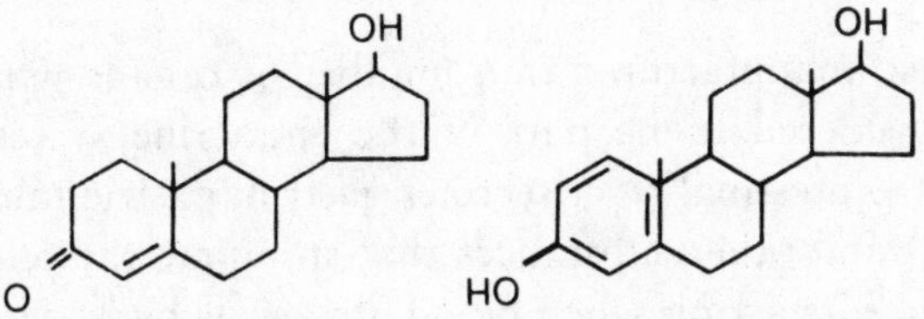

Figure 4. Chemical structure of testosterone and an oestrogen, highlighting similarities

hormones are secreted at a fairly steady rate, while a woman's follows a cyclical pattern, controlling her menstrual and fertility cycle. This book is intended to sort out fact from myth and so discussion in the area will constantly recur.

For both sexes, the production of reproductive hormones is controlled by a feedback system between the hypothalamus – pituitary axis and the gonads. In men, the pituitary hormone FSH regulates the production of sperm, while LH, also a pituitary hormone, controls secretion of testosterone. This, and other androgens are responsible for growth of the male beard, deeper voice, broad-shouldered, muscular development of a man's body. Androgens control our sexual desires and are also thought to be responsible for male aggressiveness, a greater willingness to fight, boisterousness and so on.

The female ovaries manufacture oestrogens and progesterone, as well as other hormones and a small amount of testosterone. The most important oestrogen is oestradiol, a general term that applies to the 'feminising' hormones. The oestrogens help promote breast development and the growth of the lining of the womb (endometrium) during the first phase of the menstrual cycle. Progesterone and oestrogen together prepare the uterine lining for pregnancy during the second phase. Another hormone is relaxin, which helps to facilitate delivery.

Because all these hormones are controlled by a complex and extremely sensitive feedback system, all operating hand in hand so to speak, all need to function properly or the overall system can go awry. Malnutrition, obesity, stress, illness, too much or too little body fat are some of the factors that can 'shut down' a woman's ovaries.

Other hormones

Hormones are also manufactured in a number of organs which are not generally considered to be part of the endocrine system. For example, the gastrointestinal tract secretes gastrin, gastric inhibitory polypeptide (GIP) and other substances that stimulate the release of insulin and enhance its action when blood glucose is high. The heart produces atrial naturitic factor which is thought to be instrumental in controlling blood pressure.

The kidneys

The kidneys are not normally thought to be part of the endocrine system but they are instrumental in the production of at least two important hormones – renin helps maintain blood pressure, while renal erythropoietic factor (REF) helps control the production of red blood cells in the bone marrow.

Renin's role is poorly understood, and it does not act directly on an organ or tissue, but on a protein called angiotensinogen which is formed in the liver and released into the blood. When this protein comes into contact with renin, a substance called angiotensin I is formed. This is converted to angiotensin II in the lungs and it constricts the small arteries and arterioles, thereby raising blood pressure. Angiotensin II also influences the release of aldosterone and seems to control thirst, an important factor in making sure the body gets enough fluids. A contribution to high blood pressure may be an imbalance of the renin-angiotensin-aldosterone system. But we do not know what prompts the kidneys to release renin. Organs other than the kidneys produce it too, with high levels having been found in the uterus and placenta of pregnant women and in the blood of people whose kidneys have been removed.

Erythropoietin controls the bone marrow's production of red cells. It was thought that the kidneys produced this hormone but it now appears that they secrete REF, which, together with a substance produced by the liver, makes erythropoietin. The body produces more of the latter following a serious bleeding episode when the number of blood cells has dropped. It also increases at high altitude when we need more blood cells to extract oxygen from the thinner air. As with renin, there seem to be other sources of erythropoietin than the kidneys.

The lungs also perform endocrine functions, as we have seen with angiotensin II production. In certain types of lung cancer, ACTH and other hormones are secreted which upset the body's hormonal balance.

How hormones work

Only minute amounts of hormones circulate in the blood so they require highly efficient mechanisms to act and extremely sensitive receptors. They seek out receptor sites which are programmed to recognise and receive them. Protein peptide hormones such as insulin do not enter a cell itself, so the receptor sites are located on or near target cells. When a protein hormone attaches itself to its receptor site, the latter transmits a message to the area of the target cell which is programmed to respond to the hormone. This entails activating an enzyme called adenyl cyclase, which is in the cell membrane, to become a second messenger, or 'hormone mediator', called cyclic AMP and this carries out the hormonal action.

Steroid hormones can cross the cellular membranes. So, they seek out a receptor inside the cell itself. The hormone and receptor form a smaller molecule which enters the cell nucleus and goes directly to its encoded portion of DNA. This activates specific genes to form messenger RNA and carry out the hormone's intended function. RNA and DNA carry the specific genetic information for the makeup of each woman's body.

Prostaglandins

These are a group of substances formed from fatty acids which are produced throughout the body and which are involved in a number of hormone-mediated functions. They were first discovered in semen and seminal vesicles, and, at first, were thought to be produced in the prostate, hence their name. Similar substances were then discovered in the kidneys, uterus and other organs.

Like cyclic AMP, prostaglandins have many different functions, depending on which tissues produce them and the hormones that mediate their activities. Prostaglandins may act as second messengers for certain hormones and cyclic AMP may be the third messenger.

Prostaglandins stimulate uterine contractions and may initiate labour. During menstruation they may cause uterine contractions, while excessive prostaglandin causes menstrual cramps. Other functions involving prostaglandins include blood clotting and the clustering of platelets, the inflammation process, immune responses, movement of the intestines and gastric secretion, metabolism and function of the nervous system.

The realisation that prostaglandins are involved in menstrual cramps has led to the widespread use of antagonists to prostaglandins, such as aspirin or non-steroidal anti-inflammatory drugs (NSAIDs), to treat this disorder which affects millions of women. They are also important in the treatment of arthritis and other inflammatory disorders. In another context, aspirin may now be prescribed to prevent thickening of the blood, apparently inhibiting the prostaglandins which cause the clustering of blood platelets and the formation of clots which can block blood flow to the heart or brain.

While many therapies involving prostaglandins entail blocking action, inducing labour is just the opposite. It is thought that the placenta produces prostaglandins in increasing amounts as the time of delivery approaches, somehow increasing uterine sensitivity to the hormone oxytocin. By injecting prostaglandins into the amniotic cavity or by inserting it into the cervix, uterine contractions can be induced. This is also a method for performing a late abortion.

Summing up

This has been a simplified overview of a very complex system of hormonal activity. The endocrine system is involved in virtually every body process. So when something goes wrong with one of the endocrine glands, the effects may be experienced in dozens of different ways. Fortunately this finely tuned system usually works so smoothly most of us are barely aware of it.

PART II

The Role of Hormones in the Milestones of a Woman's Life

CHAPTER TWO

The Early Growing Years

Infancy and childhood are generally believed to be the main growing years. But physical growth actually starts at fertilisation and continues when we are adults with cells replacing themselves. Dead skin is an obvious example. While growth is encoded at the time of conception, numerous circumstances may alter this intended growth pattern.

Growth is largely controlled by complex hormonal interactions with other body systems. Researchers have long debated whether our genes or our environment are more important in determining height, weight and other characteristics. Both seem to be important. Your genes may be programmed to produce a six-footer but illness or poor diet may stunt you.

Basically there are two types of growth: an increase in the number of cells (hyperplasia) and an increase in cell size (hypertrophy). Growth during the early embryonic stage of pregnancy (about the first 10 weeks after fertilisation) is mostly due to an increase in the number of cells as well as in cell size. Tissue growth is further classified by the nature of the cell populations. Some tissue is constantly renewing itself; for example the skin, blood, intestinal lining and male germ cells have a short lifespan. In contrast, static tissues such as neurons and muscle cells, normally live as long as the organism. If these tissues are injured or destroyed there is little or no regeneration, although the remaining cells may enlarge to try to compensate for what was lost. The third category is referred to as 'expanding tissue'; these are cells that normally grow to their appropriate size and then stop, although regeneration is possible if the tissue is injured or destroyed. Examples of this would be tissue in the endocrine glands, liver, kidney and lungs.

Growth before birth

Looking at growth overall, the time in the uterus shows a spurt of activity. By birth the fertilised egg has undergone 42 successive cycles of cell division and five more would be required to reach full adult size. By one year old the average baby has doubled in weight and increased height by 50 per cent. The first and second three-month periods (trimesters) of pregnancy show the greatest speed of cell multiplication and growth in size. The secretion of growth hormone is greater during sleep than when we are awake and this is why it is important for babies and children to get plenty of sleep. Since the foetus grows so much faster anyway it is important for the mother not only to remember that she is eating (and hopefully not smoking) for two, but also that she gets plenty of rest to meet the unborn baby's needs which are greater than hers. The foetus also needs to be in an emotionally settled environment – emotion- and sleep-starved children grow less well.

One Norwegian obstetrician is constantly demonstrating this to his expectant patients. Using electrical wave sensor equipment, he shows them the effect of his terrible violin playing on the foetus, which 'hears' through its mother's ears and still responds when she wears headphones to block out the sound! The foetus also responds to the mother when she listens to her favourite music. Cutting out smoking or alcohol, pre-conception, are the kinds of lifestyle changes which really benefit the future child.

The foetus's tissues, during the 10-week embryonic period, begin to form the various organ systems. The neural (nerve) tube which is formed along the backbone develops first, with the other organ systems budding off from it. The embryonic heart begins to beat at about the fourth week, with the organ systems rapidly following. By the fifth and sixth weeks, the eyes, facial features and limbs form. By weeks eight and 10 virtually all of the organ systems are formed and many are functioning. During the first few weeks of pregnancy the embryo is particularly vulnerable to X-rays, chemicals or other substances which can affect organ development. This is a period when congenital (existing from birth) defects are likely to develop, as well as hereditary defects passed on through the chromosomes from the

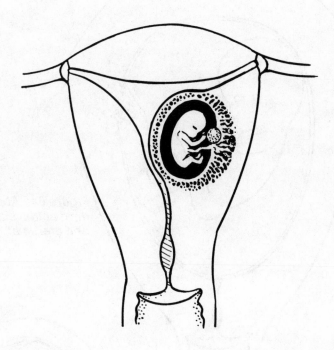

Figure 5. The actual size of the embyro and uterus at six to eight weeks

parents and grandparents. Chromosomes contain the genetic codes which are passed on from generation to generation. If a woman does not know that she is pregnant, she may take a drug or other substance which may cause her baby to be born with defects. Again, planning for two of you starts before conception, like getting into the right frame of mind and readiness for a holiday.

After the 10th week of pregnancy the foetus experiences several marked growth spurts (see Figure 6a), the most pronounced at about the 20th week. It is then adding 2.5cm (1in) a week to height; if this were kept up through a 40-week pregnancy, the baby would be more than 1.2m (4ft) tall at birth! The woman feels that, almost overnight, she can sense her baby growing rapidly, with its movements becoming stronger and more frequent, and she finds she can no longer fit into her usual clothes.

Birth weight and size are, to some degree, determined by the size of the mother. Small women tend to have smaller babies but there is no

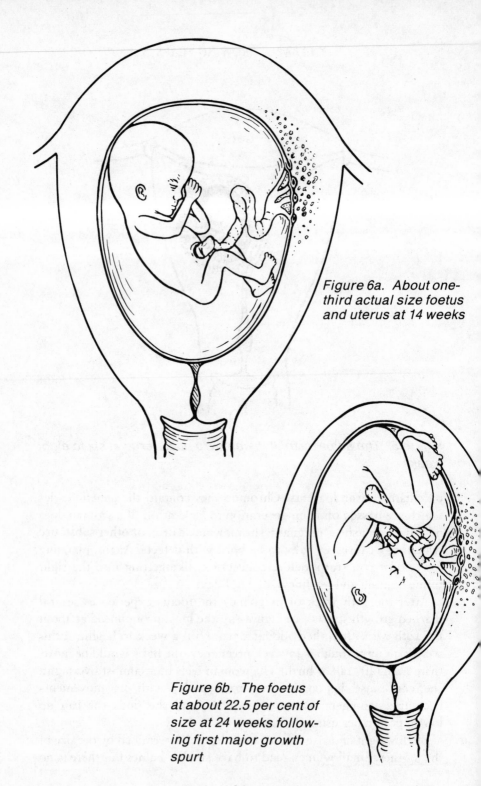

Figure 6a. About one-third actual size foetus and uterus at 14 weeks

Figure 6b. The foetus at about 22.5 per cent of size at 24 weeks following first major growth spurt

rule! A 45kg (99lb) woman, barely 1.5m (5ft) tall can have twins weighing 2.7kg to 3.1kg (6–7lb). And a tall, large-boned woman may have a tiny, full-term baby weighing less than 2.3kg (under 5lb). But then babies born to Andean women are significantly smaller than those in Lima which is at sea level, where the air has more oxygen than in the high mountains. The average birth weight of Cheyenne Indians is about 3.75kg (8lb 5oz) compared to an average birth weight of 2.4kg (5lb 4oz) for Luni tribe babies in Papua New Guinea. Environment and heredity both play a part in these cases.

For most women their first babies tend to be a few ounces lighter than later ones and boys are usually heavier than girls. In boy/girl twins the male seems to make the girl a heavier baby than if both twins were girls. Teenagers and first-time mothers over the age of 38 also seem to have smaller than average babies.

A number of hormones promote growth. Before birth, insulin and human placental lactogen are important. Some experts also take the view that an expectant mother who is diabetic, and so has high blood-sugar levels, may have a foetus which starts to make large amounts of insulin to counteract the sugar level. So the foetus grows large and may weigh 4kg (9lb) or more at birth (see Chapter 5).

Both human growth hormone (hGH), which is secreted by the pituitary, and insulin (secreted by the pancreas) play important roles too in growth after birth. A failure by the pituitary to produce adequate hGH can result in dwarfism. Calcium also comes into play because the early years of growth are when the skeleton is developing. Milk as a calcium source is well known in this context but an overall, balanced diet holds the key to growth in height and strength of the skeleton. We have already said that sleep is important because this is a time when hormone secretion increases. But it does no harm to recall the old saying that in order to grow a child needs three things: oxygen, love and a balanced diet. Children who are hypoxic (who lack adequate oxygen in the bloodstream as, for example, in certain congenital heart defects) do not grow. Emotionally deprived children and those who are not fed properly do not grow. If things do not seem right, then it is time to see whether a child's diet needs altering, for example, if they cannot tolerate milk.

After birth, thyroid hormones are needed for growth. If a child is deficient in these from the moment it is born and it goes unnoticed, then it lead to cretinism. This causes retardation, dwarfism, a large head, thick limbs, pug nose, swollen eyelids, short neck and other deformities. Mothers with a certain type of thyroid deficiency can pass this on but it can be attended to in the baby. Cretinism can be prevented by administering thyroxine at birth and it can also be given if thyroid deficiency develops later in childhood. At this older age growth may have stopped, but there is not necessarily any mental retardation. Correcting the deficiency can result in a period of speeded up growth.

The sex hormones oestrogen and androgen also promote growth. An excess of them in infancy and early childhood can result in a rapid spurt and early sexual development. If this excess is not corrected, sexual development will take place but growth will stop and children can end up abnormally short as adults (see Chapter 3).

Just as the sex hormones can stop growth, so the hormone cortisol can arrest skeletal growth by closing the bones' growth plates. Steroids, such as hydrocortisone, also affect the growth of non-renewing tissue such as skeletal muscle. The effects tend to be permanent so, if not attended to, children cannot catch up with growth as they can do if excess sex hormone production is treated. That is why this must be taken into account when steroids are proposed for juvenile arthritis, asthma or organ transplants.

While the hormones are at work, the peptides, made of amino acids, help the growth of both tissues and of tumours. Nerve growth factor is one such peptide. Platelet-derived growth factor helps heal cuts and may cause the development of atherosclerosis – the build-up of fatty deposits in the coronary and other arteries. Then there are the somatomedins, somewhat like insulin, through which growth hormone and possibly other growth factors act. Their precise role is unclear, but perhaps dwarfism is caused by a lack of them even when levels of growth hormones are normal.

Patterns of growth

Some of a baby's physical attributes can be seen in the parents and grandparents or other close relatives. However, there are many exceptions, so you cannot judge growth on family history alone. Big or small at birth, the best predictor of potential growth is assessment using growth curves. These show normal patterns of height and weight. It is important to recognise that growth is not a steady process. Parents who wonder whether a child is growing properly may be being misled by very specific, rapid spurts of growth and then the slowdowns. If a child has been progressing in keeping with the growth curve appropriate for it, and then without apparent reason starts to deviate from the pattern normal for the child itself, it may be a signal that something is wrong. Such inconsistency needs to be investigated.

Short stature

Most children who are defined as shorter than 'normal' (two or more standard deviations below the mean for their age) are in fact normal! They are simply genetically programmed to be short. However, in the case of a small number of these children there may be some other cause, and even where there is genetic shortness this may be contributed to by poor nutrition or other factors. It was once assumed that the short stature of the Japanese compared to other people in the region was a genetic characteristic. But the marked increase in stature among Japanese in the US, and among children born after World War II, seems to indicate there was a lack of calcium or something else in the Japanese diet.

So, to spot if a child has a growth problem, look back at family history, ask grandparents, see if there are records of babies further back in the family for height and weight at birthdays, or starting walking. Secondly check whether there has been a noticeable change in your child's growth pattern, because if the curve is steady and consistent without any glaring abnormalities there is probably no cause for concern. Noticeable changes should be investigated.

Most paediatricians begin to be concerned if a child drops two or more standard deviations below the average for that age group. The doctor may then do a thorough family history and a detailed physical examination to analyse the growth pattern to date. This is filled out by straightforward blood and urine tests and X-rays taken of the hand, wrist and perhaps skull to see how bone growth is going, compared to the average for that age group. Sometimes a chromosomal analysis may be performed as well as tests of growth hormone levels during sleep and in response to certain stimuli like the deliberate lowering of blood sugar.

It will be useful to look in more detail now at the growth factors of environment, hormonal abnormalities and diseases and inborn defects of bone and tissue.

Environmental factors

Worldwide, two-thirds of all children suffer from malnutrition, so it is the leading environmental cause of failure to grow and it is not confined to the Third World. The internal organs can shrink and waste (a disease called marasmus) because of a lack of calories and protein in the diet. This may be worsened by chronic diarrhoea caused by a flattening of the intestinal lining and a shortage of enzymes which help digestion. In kwashiorkor, the intake of calories may be high enough to maintain some body fat but this masks a severe lack of protein, which causes a failure to grow normally. This condition is characterised by a large, distended abdomen.

Most of us are aware of anorexia nervosa, voluntary starvation, which causes a halt in growth and this is found particularly amongst adolescent girls. Younger children may have their growth limited because their mothers do not want them to get fat. Indeed, there may be a history of anorexia nervosa in the mother's background. But, while the pre-adolescent child may stop eating out of fear of getting fat, she does not usually engage in self-induced vomiting, over-use of laxatives or excessive exercising, which adolescents may indulge in to limit weight gain. A lack of zinc or iron in the diet, or a failure by the body to absorb them can also hinder growth.

Psychosocial dwarfism is the term used to denote the failure to grow in a child that has suffered emotional deprivation, abuse or neglect. Such children often develop bizarre eating habits and have a variety of emotional problems.

Hormonal abnormalities and other diseases

Pituitary dwarfism
There are a range of problems related to a lack of growth hormone. This deficiency could be due to an abnormal pituitary gland, infections or injuries that damage it or tumours of the hypothalamus or the pituitary. Such damage can be caused by radiation treatment for a brain tumour. A rare, inherited disorder, called Laron's dwarfism makes some children resistant to growth hormone, and this is mostly in people from the Middle East when there is a history of intermarriage.

Pituitary dysfunction in children can be treated by administering growth hormone and this is now artificially synthesised. It is important to ensure that it is not derived from human sources as it was in the past, because this seemed to be linked with deaths of several youngsters from cancerous tumours.

Thyroid deficiency

Blood tests for thyroxine or thyroid-stimulating hormone can detect this deficiency in newborn babies and although this may be a routine post-natal test in countries such as the US, this is not true of every country and there are differing medical views on their necessity. Where there is a deficiency, a failure to administer adequate thyroid hormone in the first few weeks of life can cause permanent mental retardation and lead to other characteristics of cretinism.

When the thyroid does not grow properly, this does not show symptoms of an underactive thyroid and so this cause of deficiency can go unnoticed. On diagnosis and treatment, however, children usually enjoy a catch-up growth spurt.

Excessive steroids

Apart from the over-prescription of steroids, possibly causing a stop to growth (a development that cannot be reversed), tumours can sometimes produce excessive steroids. They may also result from excessive production of ACTH, which stimulates steroid production. Where steroids have to be prescribed, they can be given on an intermittent basis to minimise their effect.

Malabsorption syndrome

This is when your body does not absorb the nutrients it needs, for example if you have an intolerance to lactose (milk sugar) caused by a lack of the enzyme lactase, or an intolerance to gluten in wheat and certain breads. In such instances it is not so much a failure to grow which sparks concern, but the apathy, loss of appetite, recurrent diarrhoea and unusual stools. Treatment of lactose intolerance consists of avoiding milk and milk products. The condition is more common amongst communities of Asian or African origin. Coeliac disease is treated by avoiding gluten-containing foods. Symptoms also include a bloated stomach, anaemia and the passing of foul-smelling, fatty stools which float on the water in the toilet. If it is left to progress, it causes a flattening of the fingerlike villi which line the intestinal walls, whose job it is to absorb nutrients from the digestive tract.

Crohn's disease and other inflammatory bowel disorders
Children with inflammation of the bowel may experience slowed growth before showing signs of intestinal disorder. The causes of inflammation may be steroids, growth-inhibiting drugs which may be used to counter the inflammation and anaemia caused by internal bleeding.

Diabetes
For those diabetic children who survived for any length of time before insulin treatment became available, failure to grow was a common characteristic. But there is no shortage in height in diabetic children today because insulin replacement is available.

Mental retardation
It is common for children who are mentally retarded or who have some disorders of the central nervous system to be abnormally short. The direct cause is unknown but it may be compounded by eating disorders or a lack of growth hormone.

Kidney disease
Chronic kidney disease reduces potential for growth because of its interplay with protein intake, depletion of calcium and potassium in the body affecting bone growth, hormonal imbalances, the later development of puberty and possible use of steroids in treatment.

Heart disease
Children born with congenital heart defects may also suffer retarded growth due to inadequate oxygen or impaired blood flow.

Other disorders
Illnesses such as rickets, diseases of the body's metabolism and cancer interfere with growth, although other symptoms generally overshadow the lack of growth. A loss of weight may be the first sign of a problem.

Tall stature

People are not usually over-concerned at being taller than average though it is probably as common as being short. This may be because there are fewer disorders associated with being taller and less social stigma. However, as mentioned earlier, if excessive growth is associated with premature sexual development or abnormality in the body's proportions the cause should promptly be diagnosed and treated. Such disorders include:

Pituitary giantism
This is usually caused by a tumour that secretes growth hormone. It is a rare disorder characterised by a very rapid growth spurt and a change in features (similar to acromegaly), such as an overgrown lower jaw, a thickening of the hands and feet and an overgrowth of soft tissue. If the tumour presses upon the pituitary, then other hormonal disorders may appear. Treatment entails removing the tumour while preserving normal pituitary function. The tumour removal involves complex and delicate surgery.

Inborn errors

Premature puberty
Early onset of puberty is the most common cause of excessive growth in babies and young children. An unusual growth spurt is accompanied by signs of sexual maturity such as the growth of pubic hair, development of breasts in girls and enlargement of the penis and testes in boys. All growth will stop if this premature development is allowed to progress, so intervention is required (see Chapter 3).

Summing up

The majority of children follow an orderly pattern of growth from birth until puberty. A relatively small number are evenly divided between those taller or shorter than average, and in many cases that is due to their normal genetic programming. But environmental factors such as malnutrition or neglect, hormonal imbalances and various diseases can cause growth disorders.

CHAPTER THREE

Adolescence and Sexual Development

Adolescence is a turbulent time. Emotionally charged years, they are often as difficult for parents as for the child growing into adulthood. The child has to come to terms with sexuality, strives to achieve greater independence and tackle the psychological changes that are part of growing up.

Puberty occurs at this time through a tremendous growth spurt, sexual development and maturity. These are controlled by hormones in a fine-tuned exercise of cooperation between the endocrine glands. Puberty normally follows an orderly progression over a period of five to eight years. In girls it first begins to show with an increase in the rate of growth and a 'budding' of the breasts. From an average of 5–7.5cm (2–3in) growth a year in childhood, the child's puberty growth spurt gives a height increase of about 25 per cent and weight almost doubles in the space of two to three years.

The age at which the changes begin varies, and breast growth may be more obvious than height change, starting at any time between the ages of 8 and 13 or 14 years, perhaps accompanied by the start of pubic hair growth, though this usually follows up to a year or so later. Armpit hair growth develops somewhat later, peaking about a year after breast 'budding', and continues at a slower rate until ovulation and menstruation are established.

The beginning of menstruation, technically known as 'menarche', is often regarded as the hallmark of puberty. It can start at any time between 8 and 16 years of age, with the average age in Western industrial societies at about $12\frac{1}{2}$ years. Improved nutrition is regarded as the main factor for girls developing earlier than in the past, though the decrease of about eight months per generation this century appears to be stabilising. One often quoted study by Tanner and Frisch suggests that menarche begins when girls reach a critical body weight of about 50kg (110lb), but views differ, with some attaching importance to hormonal effects from an increase in body fat. It is known, however, that very thin girls with little body fat, such as ballet dancers or long-distance runners, have a delayed menarche.

Regular ovulation does not always coincide with menarche, often taking one or two years to become established. So many adolescents have irregular, sometimes very heavy, periods. Their bodies are producing enough hormones to cause a growth and shedding of the uterine lining but not always producing enough FSH to cause an egg to ripen and be released. It is therefore possible that early sexual intercourse may not lead to pregnancy, creating a false sense of security and lack of care about possible conception. In other cases someone may begin ovulating early and conceive early. In this context it is important that both groups should know about, and practise, contraception from the start.

Hormonal controls of puberty

The foetus has high levels of FSH, LH and GnRH (gonadotrophin-releasing hormone), especially during the first half of gestation. As the time of birth approaches, the foetus develops a negative, sex-steroid, feedback system so it does not respond to pituitary stimulation of sex hormone. During the first two years of life this feedback system matures and becomes highly sensitive to sex steroids. As a result the hypothalamus has a very low 'set point' for sex hormones throughout childhood. So, before menarche, the ovaries secrete small amounts of oestrogen and small amounts of adrenal hormones are also converted to oestrogen. The hypothalamus senses these tiny amounts and signals the ovaries to continue producing them so there is no rise in the amount of the other steroids. This would take place if the oestrogen level was to fall. As puberty approaches, this 'set point' gradually rises, and secretion of of GnRH rises too. This leads to increased production of the FSH and LH gonadotrophins, and the gonads respond by producing more sex hormones – oestrogens in girls and testosterone in boys.

43

As the feedback system changes, the level of gonadotrophins rises gradually – a phenomenon that occurs at an earlier age in girls than in boys. What prompts the changes in the hypothalamus is not known, but nerve signals may play a role. The hormonal changes are also closely related to the sleeping/waking cycle with pulses of LH, and, to a lesser degree, FSH, being secreted during sleep, and smaller amounts being released during the day. The trigger for these changes is not known, but children approaching adolescence do seem to want to sleep more, or with naps on coming home from school, even if before this they have been early risers and wanted to go to bed late. It is important for parents to realise this need for extra sleep.

Appetite also seems to perk up to the point of voraciousness, particularly in boys. The extra food provides the tremendous amount of energy needed for the growth spurt and probably helps girls achieve the weight and body proportions needed to signal the onset of menstruation. In all this the hypothalamus seems to act as the control centre, processing signals from other parts of the brain and the nervous system (see Figure 7). Different hormones influence development of secondary sex characteristics, with oestrogens in girls accounting for breast development, changes in sweat glands which produce body odour, changes in the vagina and its secretions, and enlargement of the external genitals. Androgens, which are secreted in small amounts by the ovaries and adrenal glands, control the growth of pubic and axillary hair.

The hormones responsible for the adolescent growth spurt are in some ways independent of the gonadotrophins. Youngsters who fail to develop sexually may still experience a growth spurt and vice versa. But in other respects the two are interdependent. For example, maximum growth in an adolescent girl takes place before menarche; growth slows with menarche, and when she starts ovulating and achieves adult levels of oestrogen, further growth ceases. One reason why men tend to be taller than women is that girls enter puberty earlier, while boys, who are generally taller than girls when they begin their growth spurt, continue to grow about two years longer than girls.

With the onset of puberty there is also a marked change in body composition, which differentiates the male from the female. Before puberty, lean muscle mass, bones and fat are about equal. While a girl's body takes on female contours, a boy develops more muscle mass, with males ending up not only with twice as many muscle cells

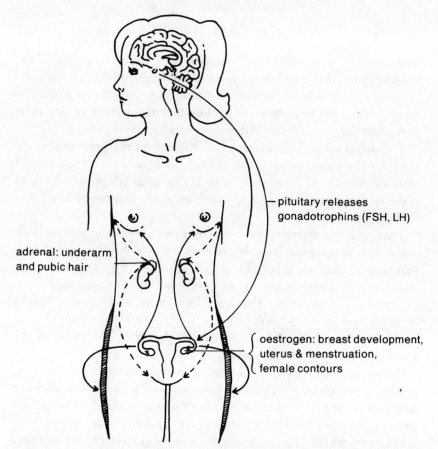

*Figure 7. How hormones initiate puberty: with the onset of
puberty, pituitary hormones stimulate the ovaries to increase
production of the female sex hormones, which in turn stimulate
development of secondary sex characteristics*

as women, but cells that are actually larger, as well as heavier bones.
In contrast the average male has less body fat (12–15 per cent of
total), while the body of an average, trim woman may have 25 per
cent of her weight in fat. This explains why men have more physical
strength than women and is one of the reasons why women experience more bone loss as they grow older, because they have less bone
mass to start with (see Chapter 6).

Psychological changes

Parents are often upset and puzzled by changes in their children's
moods during puberty, with a normally friendly child becoming

irrational and impossible from one minute to the next. Energy alternates with apathy; what their friends think of them becomes very important. Children honestly cannot explain why they feel a particular way. A clue for women is how they feel themselves before their periods as surges in certain hormones produce mood swings.

The assertion of independence at this age means pressures on all sides for the young person, not only in the home, but at school and amongst friends and enemies. It is also a time when they have to come to terms with social drugs such as alcohol, tobacco and other harmful substances.

There are also internal pressures from trying to come to terms with one's own developing sexuality, something which most parents are reluctant to discuss, especially sexual practices. Fortunately, magazines for young people provide surveys about safe sex and what sex is all about in relationships. This is a safety net for what may be lacking at home and in the school, but it may do health professionals and parents some good to read them too so that they are aware of the knowledge base of young people.

There are still many adolescent misunderstandings about sex, mainly the result of poor education on sex and sexuality. Parents can help by creating an atmosphere where there is available information (leaving the right books around can help) and also making sure both sexes know where to go to find out about contraception and safe sex, particularly in these times of AIDS. But the massive increase in sexually transmitted diseases (compared to a few decades ago and despite the fear of AIDS) is another good reason why safe sex should be familiar ground for young people. Certainly the Richard Branson Virgin empire and its sale of condoms has done a great deal to break down adult taboos to the benefit of the young. AIDS has positive spinoffs too. Adults need to understand that a young person's sensible approach to sexuality, or enjoying a drink, but not driving, is more of a priority than the kind of clothes or hairstyle which they sport. Parents must avoid missing the wood for the trees.

Delayed puberty

The failure to mature sexually due to delayed puberty is relatively rare. Usually, a girl of 13, or a boy of 14, who shows no sign of sexual development (breast budding in girls and growth of the testes and penis in boys) should be evaluated by a doctor. Some may 'bloom' late without treatment and have no obvious abnormalities, such as undescended testicles. Family history can help, revealing for example, a mother who did not start menstruating till her teens, or a father who entered puberty late. Bone X-rays may show a child is behind in growth compared to age; she may have normal sexual development later, but be shorter than average. Treatment for delayed puberty may involve use of an artificial form of GnRH, or a course of oestrogen tablets for girls or testosterone injections for boys.

Tumours, congenital defects, pituitary or thyroid disorders, malnutrition (including anorexia nervosa), serious diseases and some rare syndromes can upset hormonal function and lead to delayed puberty and so a failure to mature sexually. Where there appears to be a delay in sexual development, along the lines of what we have already said, early investigation is essential rather then waiting to further traumatise an already traumatised 17-year-old.

Tumours

While inadequate production of the correct hormones are the primary cause of rare failure to develop sexually, tumours (not necessarily malignant cancers) growing near the pituitary and hypothalamus in the brain can also cause delayed puberty. They do this by interfering with the secretion of gonadotrophins and GnRH respectively, and also with the production of growth hormone. Signs of tumours include a sudden halt in normal growth, headaches, eye trouble, weakness in the arms or legs. Diabetes insipidus, a disorder marked by thirst, dehydration and excessive production of urine, also may be caused by a pituitary tumour that interferes with the production of vasopressin, the hormone that helps maintain the body's fluid balance, rather than getting rid of body fluid.

Some tumours can actually produce their own hormones (eg prolactin) and so knock out the body's balance, but they are usually seen in older teenagers. Overproduction of prolactin can stop menstruation in a girl even though she has developed normally through puberty. It stimulates the breast to make milk. That is why breastfeeding acts as a contraceptive in breastfeeding mothers. Interestingly both girls and boys can begin to produce milk if they start to produce an excess of prolactin. Suspected tumours are usually easy to confirm with a brain scan and treatment by a variety of techniques is possible.

Pituitary disorders

In the rare Kallman syndrome the pituitary does not secrete the hormones which trigger the production and release of gonadotrophins. Boys may have undescended testicles, girls do not develop breasts and both lack their normal male and female characteristics. There may also be associated congenital defects such as cleft lip, cleft palate, epilepsy and an impaired sense of smell.

In pituitary dwarfism the defect may be isolated growth hormone deficiency. Sexual development occurs and this stops the child reaching full height if not diagnosed and treated before puberty.

Thyroid disorders

An underactive thyroid (hypothyroidism), resulting in a deficiency of thyroid hormones, may cause delayed puberty or halt periods in a woman who has already entered the menarche. While the problem may lie in the thyroid gland itself, it could also be the pituitary failing to produce the hormone whose job it is to signal the thyroid to produce its own hormones. Treatment with the appropriate hormones usually solves the problem.

Severe hypothyroidism may, paradoxically, cause a converse effect, premature puberty. If the thyroid is not working properly the pituitary may go into overtime; it produces large amounts of thyrotropin-releasing factor to get the thyroid to produce its own hormones. It seems that this stimulates the secretion of gonadotrophins and prolactin, leading to an early onset of puberty and the production of breastmilk. Treatment is with thyroid hormone.

Malnutrition

Anorexia nervosa is one of the more common causes of delayed or interrupted puberty among girls in Western society. A life-threatening disorder, the person affected becomes so obsessed with body image and thinness that she resorts to self-starvation. The problem may be masked by a preoccupation with some physical activity, such as running or ballet dancing.

It mainly affects adolescent girls or young women. The cause is unclear, although some point to the hypothalamus which houses the appetite centre. There does seem to be a combination of factors, with many victims being very bright, feeling driven to succeed and be in control, and coming from middle- or upper-class families where too much store is set by certain standards of behaviour and achievement.

The eating problem usually begins with the onset of puberty and for this reason some suggest it is connected with a youngster's fear of menstruation and the pressure of assuming adult responsibilities.

Often the parents are not aware of the eating problem until it reaches an advanced stage. Behind a facade of normal eating, the youngster may secretly force herself to vomit or use diuretics or laxatives to weigh less. It may become apparent if the girl has started to menstruate and then stops or menstruates infrequently. This is caused by a loss of weight, which gives a signal to the body to stop producing the hormones needed to stimulate the ovaries. In its own way this is a normal protective mechanism through which the body, sensing it is being starved, takes action to conserve as much energy as possible. All metabolism slows down, and the body starts to convert protein in muscles and so forth into energy. It is converting lean body tissue and muscle cells for this purpose and so the muscles begin to waste and there is dangerous loss of heart muscle. Despite the appearance to others of a concentration camp victim, the girl will maintain she is too fat. Untreated, a large percentage of victims will succumb to starvation. Hospitalisation and artificial feeding are temporary measures to counter this but relapses are common. The most useful approach has been a combination of individual psychotherapy, family therapy and group treatment with other anorexics. Any solution is a long-term one.

There are unfortunately more cases than there should be of parental neglect of children which leads to malnutrition. Particular care needs to be taken by parents today where school meals have been pared back or are not taken because of cost, or because children 'eat out' at lunchtime because they are not attracted to the school menu. This is not the place to discuss 'junk' food but its role in a balanced diet needs to be watched, because the way the body is maintained and 'serviced' through childhood is the way it will be for life.

Precocious puberty

This can be as disturbing as delayed puberty; it affects about six in every thousand. The signs of puberty appear before the age of about nine in boys and eight in girls. In newborn babies it shows in tiny breasts and enlarged genitals because of high levels of sex hormones in the mother during pregnancy. But these soon disappear and the body becomes normal. When it occurs in a child however, this 'sexual infantilism' persists until puberty. Unusually, a child may inherit a tendency for what is called constitutional precocious puberty and this may be seen from its family's history.

Early puberty is that which develops at the age of eight or nine for boys and seven or eight for girls. Generally it has a number of identifiable causes including tumours affecting the hypothalamus. The tumour can interfere with the normal feedback system which keeps the hormone balance, leading to a premature rise in gonadotrophins and producing an early onset of puberty.

Surgery is often difficult because of the location of the tumours in the brain and radiation therapy is sometimes used for treatment. Other factors that can lead to early puberty: encephalitis (inflammation of the brain), brain abscesses, infections, head injuries and brain cysts.

Other causes

Disorders in the central nervous system have been associated with early puberty such as McCune-Albright syndrome and von Recklinghausen's disease. Both are characterised by brownish 'cafe-au-lait' spots on the body. Children with von Recklinghausen's disease (neurofibromatosis) also have overgrowth of the sheaths encasing the nerves and other fibrous tissue. Eye trouble, seizures and mental retardation are common characteristics. Delayed puberty is possible.

Steroid drugs during infancy or early childhood may sometimes cause early puberty by stimulating an overgrowth of the adrenal glands and overproduction of adrenal hormones. Care should also be taken to make sure that children do not accidentally swallow adult hormone therapy drugs, or any cosmetic preparations containing hormones. Overdosing on these could cause a young girl to ingest enough oestrogen to stimulate her own ovaries and so increase hormone production. Boys receiving hCG, a gonad-stimulation preparation to treat undescended testes, may start puberty early because of testosterone produced in the process.

Puberty may also be incomplete; in such situations a little girl may develop breasts and perhaps pubic hair This is most commonly caused by increased oestrogen production, usually from a small cyst on an ovary, or more rarely from an oestrogen-producing tumour. But the changes will reverse or stop with onset of menstruation.

Occasionally girls up to the ages of three or four have breast enlargement that persists for several months and then recedes. This may be caused by an ovarian cyst or a rise in follicle-stimulating hormone. In very rare instances a hormone-producing tumour can produce characteristics of the opposite sex and this is a very serious disorder.

Boys approaching puberty may experience breast development, perhaps caused by excessive oestrogen but this usually resolves itself as puberty progresses and muscle development occurs.

Precocious puberty can be disturbing for children and parents because the child may have adult sexual characteristics in contrast to their social and intellectual development. In most cases early puberty is treated with compensatory hormone treatment.

Associated with abnormal puberty are the Prader-Willi and the Laurence-Moon-Biedl syndromes. Particular to the latter is the eye disorder retinitis pigmentosa, and both are characterised by massive obesity, shortness and mental retardation.

Gonadal disorders

Sometimes chromosomal and congenital defects affect puberty. Babies may be born without ovaries, testes or full reproductive systems, or there may be a crossover with a child having female genitalia yet lacking proper female chromosomes.

At one in 500, Klinefelter's syndrome is the most common abnormality; it causes small, hard testes, impaired sperm production, men perhaps looking like eunuchs, with a small penis, developed breasts, little or no body hair and serious psychological problems.

In girls, Turner's syndrome is the most common gonadal malformation, characterised by failure to mature sexually, short stature and a variety of birth defects, depending on the chromosomal pattern. But this is much rarer than Klinefelter's syndrome.

Summing up

Most children move naturally from childhood to adulthood. Emotional changes are usually more difficult to handle than the physical ones but an open mind, mutual respect and understanding and a sense of humour help to get most families through adolescence.

CHAPTER FOUR

The Menstrual Cycle

Through the ages menstruation has been viewed with a mixture of awe and distaste – an attitude that continues to plague women throughout the world. It is surprising how many misconceptions still persist.

In primitive societies, magical properties were often ascribed to menstruation and they rightly thought blood was vital to life. For a woman to bleed without any lasting danger was awesome. Many cultures considered menstrual blood and menstruating women unclean and they were often kept apart during menstruation. This was so they could not contaminate others or exercise their magic. They believed a menstruating woman could ruin crops, make cows go dry, turn milk or wine sour, cause natural disasters and summon demons to possess a person.

Religions have evolved practices and taboos which may still govern menstruation and childbirth. The Bible contains the laws of Moses, which indicated that a menstruating woman was unclean, as was everything she touched. Sex was forbidden during, and for a week after, menstruation. The man was not to come into contact with her or anything she had touched, even the chair she had sat on. This led to segregation in public places lest a man accidentally came into contact with an 'unclean' woman.

But practical reasons may have led to the customs that governed sexual behaviour. A better chance of conception, for example, is likely to follow abstinence, so some societies have thought the start of the fertile days after menstruation increased opportunity, especially for conceiving a male child. The Israelites needed to increase their population and ensuring sex took place during the fertile part of the month was one way of achieving this. During the wandering in the desert there were a number of laws on hygiene, including those relating to food, to keep risks of infection low, particularly because of the lack of water for cleaning and washing.

Despite modern education, menstruation is still popularly seen as 'being sick'. The unclean connotation has been grafted onto phrases such as 'sanitary' towels. In fact, menstrual blood is sterile and odourless until exposed to the air. Because there is no sickness or weakness through injury, there is no reason why menstruating women should not exercise and carry out physical tasks, unless of course they have cramps or bleed heavily. Old wives' tales are more of a social hindrance rather than the result of medical fact.

Women's perceptions and experience of menstruation vary widely. Some feel unwell, suffering from cramps, headaches and other symptoms. Others may be irritable, nervous and emotionally out-of-kilter at specific times during their menstrual cycle. Yet other women experience neither physical or psychological effects.

Some women menstruate every 27 to 30 days. Others are erratic, with two or three periods close together and then a couple of months until the next one. Some menstruate for two or three days, others for five or six, with the flow ranging from scanty to heavy. So it is a highly individualistic phenomenon. Many women worry needlessly that they are different when, in fact, there is no clear 'average' and this is not helped because they are reluctant to talk to their doctors.

Hormonal controls

Menstruation is the regular shedding of a portion of the tissue that lines the uterus. During the early part of the cycle, this lining – the endometrium – grows, becomes thicker and enriched with blood vessels in preparation to receive a fertilised egg and establish a pregnancy. When conception does not take place the lining stops growing and the surface two-thirds of the endometrium breaks down, because it is no longer needed, and is shed through the vagina. About half to three-quarters of the menstrual fluid is blood, the rest being made up of cells, mucus and bits of the lining membrane.

The uterus produces an enzyme which destroys some of the clotting factors normally found in blood and this is why menstrual blood does not clot. What seem to be clots are more likely to be

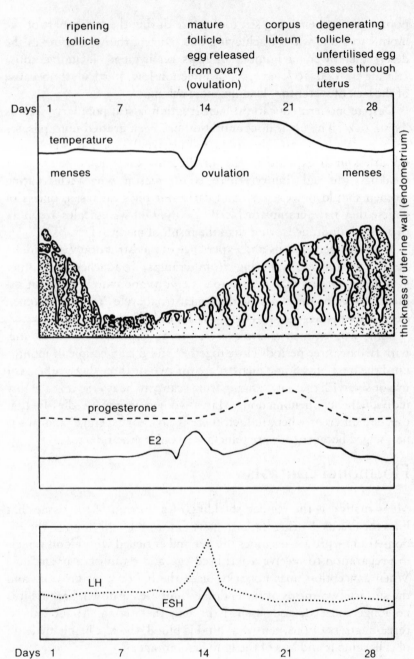

Figure 8. The menstrual cycle

clumps of cells and other material shed from the lining of the uterus. If the flow is very heavy, some clots may form in the vagina after the blood has left the uterus. During an average period, only four to six tablespoons of blood are shed (the amount varying from woman to woman) but the volume seems greater because it contains other fluids and material, so women think they are losing considerably more.

The menstrual cycle graphically shows the complex relationship between various hormones. The endocrine, and often other organ systems must function properly to ensure normal cycles. Thyroid disorders can cause menstrual irregularities or stop periods. Stress, extremes in weight, certain drugs and infections are a few of the factors that can upset the cycle. This sensitivity to different factors is a protection mechanism to make sure a baby is conceived in a healthy body. Both negative and positive feedback systems come into play to regulate the cycle, working over something like a 28-day cycle (see Figure 8).

Days 1–5: the menstrual phase
Oestrogen and progesterone are at low levels, signalling the the hypothalamus and pituitary to begin secreting their trigger hormones, LH and FSH, which tell the ovaries to start a new reproductive cycle. FSH stimulates the development of a follicle within the ovary and triggers the maturation of an egg to be released on ovulation, while LH stimulates the ovaries to produce oestrogen (E2 on Figure 8).

Days 6–12: the proliferative/follicular phase
LH and oestrogen levels continue to rise, oestrogen producing a negative feedback to tell the pituitary to reduce its production of FSH but produce more LH.

Days 12–13: the proliferative phase
Oestrogen production surges, causes a corresponding increase in LH. After ovulation (below) oestrogen falls, with a corresponding rise in FSH.

Day 14: ovulation
Within 36 hours of this LH surge the follicle releases its mature egg and ovulation normally takes place. The finger-like fimbriae of the fallopian tubes grasp it and it begins to be moved down towards the uterus. If intercourse takes place, and a sperm can swim far enough,

it will unite with the travelling egg to produce fertilisation. After ovulation the ruptured follicle which produced the matured egg turns into the corpus luteum, a structure which has a new job of producing progesterone to help the uterus get ready a lining, over about 14 days, which can welcome a fertilised egg to develop a pregnancy.

Days 15–27: the luteal phase
During this second half of the cycle, progesterone continues to rise and FSH drops to its lowest level during the cycle. There is also a sharp drop in LH following ovulation, and this hormone also falls to its lowest level. The rising progesterone, peaking at about day 22 if fertilisation does not take place, changes the top layer of the uterus lining quite a lot. It doubles in thickness, its glands fill with fat and glycogen to provide food for an embryro if a fertilised egg arrives. If it does not then the corpus luteum has no job to fulfil so it starts to shrink and progesterone production drops. The lining begins to break down and loosen and by about day 27 oestrogen, progesterone, FSH and LH are at their lowest levels.

Day 28: menstruation begins and makes way for a new cycle.
We have described a hypothetical progression through the cycle because no woman operates so precisely; the average cycle is 25-30 days, with variants ranging from 20-40 days – all being normal. Whatever the length of the cycle, ovulation usually takes place about 14 days before menstruation. So, if you have a 20-day cycle you will ovulate on about day 7, and a 40-day cycle on about day 26. It is wrong, therefore, to assume that ovulation takes place midway between periods. The proliferative phase may vary in length, but the luteal phase is generally constant at about 14 days in length.

Women with a regular cycle of about 28 days may think they are irregular because they do not match the months on a wall calendar. In fact they are following a lunar calendar, so they could have 13 periods in the year. Use a calendar, of course, to keep track of your periods.

Problems related to menstruation

There is debate and controversy about how different hormonal changes affect the way a woman behaves and feels during the cycle, much of it coloured by what, for long, has been a male-dominated medical profession. Regretfully, even now there have been recent instances where some doctors still associate mental illness with some of the effects of menstruation.

Physical discomfort

Many women experience swelling of the abdomen, ankles, feet and fingers, aching joints, muscle stiffness, feelings of heaviness and acne. The swelling and aches may be connected with oestrogen causing salt and water retention but acne should improve with oestrogen not worsen, so the picture is not clear. Breasts may swell after menstruation starts and some women keep two sizes of bra. But it may be very uncomfortable for women with benign cystic disease because the cysts accumulate fluid and swell. Cramps and diarrhoea around the start of menstruation may be due to prostaglandins rather than changes in steroid hormone levels, though some think a role is played by increased levels of progesterone. In contrast some women suffer from constipation (it may alternate with diarrhoea). For women suffering from migraine or vascular headaches in the pre-menstrual phase, the tiny muscles which control the circumference of blood vessels may be oversensitive to the high levels of steroids. Headaches can be caused by the expansion of the arteries in the head, followed by a contraction of the vessels. Some women find that their varicose veins swell and ache, and others experience episodes of rapid heartbeats.

Mood swings are common, with difficulties in sleeping, restlessnes and fatigue, accompanied by tetchiness with others around them who do not make allowances. Studies have found that pre-menstrual women are more likely to be involved in accidents.

Another facet of the cycle is craving for food, particularly sweets or salty food, and while some women become ravenous, others lose their appetite. Some become thirsty while others are more affected by alcohol than usual. It is useful to use the checklist (see Table 1), and see where, if at all, you find any similarities with your own cycle.

Pre-menstrual syndrome or tension (PMT) is a term used when these changes become incapacitating. As already mentioned, until recently these symptoms were regarded by many doctors as psychological. The most significant change in understanding began in the 1950s when Dr Katherine Dalton in the UK published the results of her studies on the menstrual cycle, detailing symptoms associated with the pre-menstrual phase. This put the work of a number of ignored researchers on the map.

Table 1: Common symptoms of pre-menstrual tension

General

Altered sex drive
Swelling, especially of abdomen, feet and ankles
Breast swelling and pain
Dizziness
Fatigue
Increased hunger, food cravings, especially for sweets/savouries
Insomnia
Headaches, often vascular or migraine
Muscular or joint pain
Tendency to low blood sugar (hypoglycaemia)
Palpitations
Restlessness
Ringing in the ears
Swollen or aching varicose veins
Thirst
Urinary frequency
Weight gain

Gastrointestinal

Bowel cramps
Constipation
Diarrhoea
Nausea
Vomiting

Psychological

Anxiety
Crying spells
Depression
Irritability
Mood swings

Whatever the climate of opinion in the past, your menstrual cycle and any PMT are subjects that you should have no hestitation in raising with your doctor. If you find that your doctor is unsympathetic or is not up to date with possible treatments, then you should consider asking for referral to someone else, or if the situation with your own doctor becomes difficult, then consider changing the doctor. The problem is that insufficient research has been done in this field to develop specific treatments or understanding of causes, so doctors do not necessarily have answers, even if they keep abreast of what have been slow developments in this field. However, where there is excessive swelling, reducing salt and increasing potassium intake, which helps excrete fluid, may be of some benefit. But be careful because it could lead to degrees of dehydration which could upset the body's fluid and chemical balance and so upset its metabolism.

Common sense and self-help can go a long way to easing your own particular discomforts. If breasts are swollen and tender then avoid breast stimulation and wear a larger size bra which nevertheless gives adequate support. Wear looser clothes, avoid alcohol, re-schedule your day so your workload peaks when you are most at ease and make sure your diet is right and you get enough rest.

Coping with mood swings may be more difficult, but understanding what they are is the first step in tackling them, and you can then plan for them. Deep-breathing exercises as part of a relaxation strategy, meditation, keep-fit exercises can all help to reduce stress. If coffee or other regular beverages make you nervous, avoid them or drink decaffeinated. In some instances beta-blockers (propanolol) are prescribed to tackle vascular headaches but these can have side effects such as dizziness or lethargy, so they may only be a partial solution.

Hormonal treatments for PMT remain controversial. While Dr Dalton has advocated progesterone to treat severe PMT, and it helps some women, others get no benefit, so some argue it has no role to play. Some doctors prescribe progesterone in suppository form and it may help some women, particularly if given before the time when the symptoms normally show themselves. Similar uncertainty surrounds the suppression of high levels of prolactin with drugs. Some women suffer side effects from the drug bromocriptine. It may ease breast swelling and pain for women with severe fibrocystitis.

Tackling problems through diet has shown poor results. Large doses of vitamin A are claimed by some to relieve fibrocystitis in some women, but should not be taken without guidance from your doctor.

Other vitamins show no convincing effect and indeed too much vitamin A can be toxic.

Some researchers suggest PMT may spring from changes in the body's metabolism, and some studies have found an increase in insulin receptors during the latter half of the menstrual cycle which may account for lower blood sugar. Some PMT symptoms have been put down to hypoglycaemia, in particular fatigue, nervousness, perspiring, lightheadedness and increased hunger, particularly for sweet things. Some doctors recommend a diet high in complex carbohydrates in the premenstrual phase, based on the theory that it will counter low blood sugar, but there is no evidence to support this. If you know you are on a balanced diet then, of course, that can help you eliminate poor nutrition as a possible suspect.

Do not be put off – if you feel things are not right then they probably are not, and you need to hold your ground and examine all the possibilities with a sympathetic doctor, as we said before.

Menstrual cramps

Menstrual cramps, technically dysmenorrhoea, are common but treatment can now provide relief for millions because the cause of the cramps can be identified.

In about 5 to 10 per cent of women the pain has specific causes such as inflammation of the endometrium, fibroids, etc. and pain should go when these are treated. But for the majority of women there is no clear cause and this is known as primary dysmenorrhoea.

For centuries women have resorted to various treatments – heatpads, painkillers, bed rest, exercise and various herbal remedies but with no clear effect. Many doctors have turned to tranquillisers such as diazepam (Valium), arguing the pain is largely psychologically-based. But now the use of non-steroidal anti-inflammatory drugs (NSAIDs), used to treat arthritis, may be effective for a high proportion of women. They block the production or action of prostaglandins. Menstrual blood contains high levels of these and they help to cause uterine contractions. But their role in menstrual cramps is not clear. Some studies suggest a high level of prostaglandins causes excessive contractions of the uterine muscles, so clamping the blood vessels and in turn causing pain because the flow of oxygen to the muscles is reduced. During pregnancy, the number of blood vessels supplying the uterus increases and some of these remain after childbirth. So, even though the uterine muscle may still contract during menstruation, there is enough circulation of oxygen-carrying blood to hold off pain from oxygen starvation. This may explain why many women cease to experience dysmenorrhoea following childbirth. But this does not explain why some women who never had cramps before childbirth, experience them after it, nor why pregnancy seems to have little effect one way or the other.

Drugs to help with dysmenorrhoea (NSAIDs) include aspirin (mild) ibuprofen (stronger), diffunisal, fenoprofen, idomethacin, mefanamic acid, naproxen, sulindac and tolmetin sodium. Side effects are common and so consultation on the use of NSAIDs is essential. Furthermore, different drugs work for different women so guidance is important. Some people are hypersensitive to aspirin and overuse may cause internal bleeding. Other NSAIDs do not usually have this particular side effect, but can cause nausea, heartburn, stomach ulcers, bloody or tarry stools (indicating intestinal bleeding), rashes, kidney irritation, sleepiness, ringing in the ears and changes in mood. These side effects are rare, especially at a low dosage, but if they occur you should stop taking the drug and advise your doctor. The approach often recommended is to take NSAIDs at the first sign of a period and not wait until the cramps strike full force. Some doctors say that the drug should be taken a day or two before menstruation. On the average, only three to six tablets are required per cycle – this is low enough to prevent the side effects that are more common in arthritis patients who may take NSAIDs several times a day over a prolonged period.

Dysmenorrhoea usually occurs only among women who are ovulating. This explains why some some young women do not experience it when they first start having periods, but begin to suffer severe cramps several months, or even a couple of years later. (It often takes up to two years for ovulation to become established.)

Women who take birth control pills usually find they no longer have menstrual cramps because the pills suppress ovulation, and though women may continue to bleed periodically this is not true menstruation. Before NSAIDs were used, oral contraceptives were often prescribed to treat cramps. Women using the pill therefore gain the benefit.

Dysfunctional bleeding
The technical phrase for any vaginal bleeding which occurs in the absence of ovulation is dysfunctional uterine bleeding. It may

coincide with and be very similar to normal menstrual periods. More often, however, the bleeding is irregular and may be heavier than in normal menstruation. Causes include tumours, both benign, such as fibroids, or cancerous ones, and hormonal imbalances in which ovulation does not place – referred to as anovulatory cycles.

Table 2: Recommended Daily Iron Intake (Mg per Day)
      (World Health Organization)

Children up to 9 years	5–10
Boys	
10–12 years	5–10
13–15	9–18
16–19	5–9
Girls	
10–12 years	5–10
13–15	12–24
16–19	24–28
Adult men (moderately active)	5–9
Adult women (moderately active)	14–28

Notes: The lower level is applicable when 25 per cent of the calories in the diet are derived from animal foods. The higher figure is necessary when animal foods make up less than 10 per cent of calories.

Pregnant women: for those whose iron intake has been at the above recommended level for a moderately active woman before pregnancy, the intake should remain the same. If, however, the iron status is not satisfactory at the beginning of pregnancy, extra iron should be taken.

Anovulatory cycles occur most often in young women who are just beginning menstruation and in older women who are approaching menopause. Oestrogen stimulates the endometrium to grow in the

Table 3: Iron Content of Foods (Mg per 100g)

Wheat germ	10.0
Bread with wheat germ	4.5
White bread	1.7
Liver, pig's stewed	17.0
Kidney, lamb's fried	12.0
Steak, lean grilled	3.4
Beefburgers, fried	3.1
Leg of lamb, lean	2.7
Leg of pork, lean	1.3
Chicken, dark meat	1.9
Chicken, white meat	0.6
Cockles	26.0
Sardines	2.4
Haddock, fried	1.2
Cod, baked	0.4
Parsley, fresh	8.0
Haricot beans, boiled	2.5
Lentils, cooked	2.4
Processed peas, canned	1.5
Spring greens, boiled	1.3
Swede, boiled	1.1
Chips	0.6
Apricots, dried	4.1
Figs, dried	2.2
Raisins	1.6
Avocado pears	1.5
Apricots, fresh	0.4
Almonds	4.2
Brazils	2.8
Hazel nuts	1.1

typical proliferative phase of the menstrual cycle. But, if ovulation does not occur, no corpus luteum forms and, without the progesterone it produces, the endometrium does not enter its second secretory stage. Instead, it continues to grow, and when oestrogen levels fall, the endometrium is shed. Such periods tend to be irregular, often with only a few days between them, and heavier than normal. So, many young girls may menstruate every two or three weeks and experience very heavy bleeding; the same is true of older women who are entering the menopause. These episodes are referred to as metrorrhagia, and since too much blood may be lost it is important to get extra iron to prevent anaemia. The best way is through your ordinary diet by ensuring you get iron-rich foods (see Table 3). But check with your doctor in case you need an iron supplement. There is a danger of going too far in the other direction and causing iron-poisoning.

An older woman who experiences irregular, heavy periods should see her doctor to rule out the possibility of cancer or a benign tumour. Of course the main reason will be that the bleeding heralds the onset of menopause. But since the chance of uterine and other reproductive cancer rises with age, it is wiser to have a check. Keeping a basal temperature chart will help a woman confirm that she is not ovulating. But of course any irregular bleeding requires investigation. This may involve taking a sample of the lining of the womb (an endometrial biopsy) and carrying out an examination under anaesthetic (dilatation and curettage).

Treatment for metrorraghia can be by hormones where no other underlying cause is diagnosed. Oestrogens and a progestogen may be given, in a form somewhat similar to the contraceptive pill. The aim of the treatment is to promote a more normal shedding of the endometrium.

Amenorrhoea – failure to menstruate
Many women and young girls are worried when they do not menstruate; this lack of periods accounts for many more questions to doctors and referrals to hospitals than heavy bleeding. Where menstruation never starts it may be called primary amenorrhoea, and secondary where menstruation has started but stops at a later time in life. But the cause could be the same. Some are self-evident: chromosomal and other abnormalities at birth including being born without ovaries or a uterus, pregnancy, hysterectomy, menopause and a completely intact hymen.

Primary amenorrhoea

Usually it is a matter of patience when an adolescent girl has not started to menstruate when most of her friends have. The age range for start of menstruation runs from 10 to 16, as explained in Chapter 3, so it is a wide variation.

The causes of a failure to menstruate (whether for the first time, or stopping after you have begun) can overlap, but Table 4 lists primary and secondary cases.

Table 4: Amenorrhoea
Causes of Primary Amenorrhoea

Lack of sufficient body fat caused by nutritional deficiency, weight loss, anorexia nervosa, athletic training disease
Hormonal disorders, including tumours of the hypothalamus and pituitary
Congenital abnormalities, including lack of ovaries or uterus
Chromosomal abnormalities
Completely intact hymen
Thyroid disease
Hormone-producing tumours or cancers
Diseases affecting the central nervous system
Diabetes, infection, other chronic diseases

Causes of Secondary Amenorrhoea

Pregnancy
Menopause
Breastfeeding
Stress
Post-pill amenorrhoea
Weight loss
Athletic training
Obesity
Hormone-producing tumours or cancers
Thyroid disease
Hormonal imbalances
Hysterectomy
Destruction of endometrium by radiation or excessive curettage
Diabetes or other chronic diseases

Drug or alcohol addiction
Adrenal disorders
Pituitary tumour or insufficiency
Ovarian cysts or tumours
Radiation
Side effect of cancer chemotherapy and other drugs
Infection

While menstruation can start, on average at up to 16 years of age, if a girl at 13 or 14 is 'flat up and down' and shows no sign of secondary sex hair, breast development etc, and there is perhaps significant family history, then investigations should not be delayed.

Pregnancy and menopause are often overlooked as obvious causes of failure to menstruate. If you have had intercourse, then go for a pregnancy test. Teenagers should remember that their doctor must treat any request for medical advice in total confidence. If you do not want to go to the family doctor you could always ring up a family planning clinic, which you can find in the phone book and where you do not necessarily have to pay for a pregnancy test.

Breastfeeding your baby normally stops menstruation for several months because high levels of prolactin suppress ovulation. But it is not guaranteed that you will not conceive if you have unprotected intercourse so contraception is needed if you are spacing your children.

Some women do not realise they have entered menopause and this is discussed in Chapter 6.

The number of causes of amenorrhoea shows how sensitive women's bodies are to all the balancing factors. Pinpointing the specific cause may need a lot of time and patience, particularly on the part of your doctor! Stress because of starting a new job, a first year at college, getting married or divorced, fear of becoming pregnant or not becoming pregnant, rape or being involved in a disaster are all examples of causes. There are many ways of tackling stress including self-help groups for yoga, relaxation and of course if you need counselling this may be arranged through your GP. You should also examine whether you are over-dieting and going below the level of fat your body needs to function normally, as we have already discussed. We know that anorexic women may stop menstruation but so also may obese women. The excessive body fat converts adrenal hormones to oestrogen, suppressing ovulation – working like oestrogen contraceptive pills.

A blocked cervix or vagina, due to an abnormal hymen or scar tissue from an infection or injury can block menstruation. The flow is blocked and reabsorbed by the body. Normal periods are re-established by surgically opening the cervix or vagina.

Endocrine disorders such as cysts on the ovaries, thyroid disorders, pituitary failure or tumours and certain cancers which produce hormones can stop menstruation.

While certain drugs can stop menstruation, the most common example is the contraceptive pill. Combination pills made up of synthetic oestrogen and progestogen maintain a constant level of sex hormones to suppress ovulation. These are normally taken for 21 days followed by no pills or placebos, containing nothing, for seven days. This stoppage usually causes the lining of the uterus to be shed. The periods which ensue maybe lighter than usual, although it is not common for them to stop altogether.

Pills which contain only progestogen usually do not suppress ovulation although the actual process is quite complicated; this includes changes which stop a fertilised egg being implanted in the lining of the uterus. That is why their effectiveness is reduced when a woman fails to take them for a few days – these pills do need to be taken continuously and without a break.

The lower dose contraceptive pills available today are less likely to cause side effects in normal women. It still needs to be said, however, that the so-called experts still seem to come up with very differing opinions, whether about heart disease, breast cancer or other risks. However, many women find that when they stop taking the pill, ovulation and menstruation may take longer to start again than they might like or expect. Most women start again within three or four months, some taking up to six months. If you're anxious to become pregnant and not wait so long, hormone treatment may help to 'wake up' the ovaries so they start producing the hormones needed to ripen and release mature eggs.

Failure to menstruate normally after coming off the pill seems to be greatest amongst thin women, who have had irregular periods in the past or who started to menstruate late. There are different viewpoints on what kind of contraception they should use. Some doctors may advise them to go for an intrauterine device (IUD) which prevents pregnancy in various 'mechanical' ways. However, for women who intend to have children at some stage, permanent infertility from the pill is very rare, whereas IUDs carry a bigger risk of inflammation of

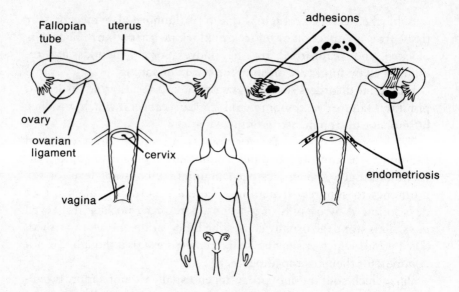

Figure 9. What happens in endometriosis: even very small clumps of endometriosis on an ovary can cause infertility. Similarly, adhesions caused by endometriosis can twist reproductive organs into abnormal shapes and prevent conception.

the tubes, which carry eggs from the ovaries, and this can block them, so causing infertility.

Psychotropic drugs to cause mood changes can affect the ovaries while they are being taken. Some chemotherapy agents, radiation therapy and indeed overexposure to X-rays can damage the ovaries. This is why, even for ordinary X-rays, lead shields should be given to adults and children to protect reproductive organs in the body. If you think you may be pregnant you should point this out to the radiographers. Always make sure you have adequate protection.

Tobacco consumption may also cause amenorrhoea, especially in thin women, and so may poor diet and alcohol.

Keeping a good diary, not just of dates but also of your general lifestyle and the way you eat, drink and exercise is probably the best source of information for the detective work which you and your doctor may need to do if you suspect there is a problem.

Endometriosis
Endometriosis is the abnormal growth, in other parts of the

68

abdomen, of tissue that normally lines the uterus. It is quite common and is a major cause of infertility, menstrual pain, abnormal bleeding, painful intercourse and other symptoms. Its cause is unknown; one theory is that the cells which cause it are formed during the embyronic stage, but when it comes to their being shed from the body there is no mechanism to trigger their release. They heal and go through the same process again and again, leading to scarring and build up around the reproductive organs. This can twist the uterus out of shape, and stop eggs being released from the ovaries into the fallopian tubes. Sometimes these cell clusters grow quite large or form dark brown, blood-filled cysts on the ovaries.

A woman may have the condition without experiencing any symptoms, and in others the pain it causes may be mistaken for menstrual cramps. The pain often begins even before menstruation starts and continues longer than most menstrual cramps, and gets worse as a woman gets older. It may take several years for the tissue to reach a painful degree and so women who have this condition may not experience the effects until they are in their early twenties. The symptoms are not necessarily related to the size of the build-up because sometimes very tiny cell clusters can produce effects as severe as those the size of an egg or larger.

Specific areas of the abdomen may become tender and a particular sexual position may be painful through pressing on a certain spot. Build-ups near the rectum or bladder may cause constipation or pain when going to the toilet. The symptoms may seem similar to pelvic inflammatory disease (PID), a potentially serious infection of the reproductive organs.

Endometriosis can also make it difficult to conceive, and we have become more aware of the condition because more women have delayed having their first child till their thirties, when endometriosis may be well established. The increased number of periods in women generally (compared to the situation generations ago) also means there is potential for more tissue growth. The abnormal tissue seems to have less time to establish itself when woman had babies at an early age and probably went through, perhaps, six pregnancies. Endometriosis almost disappears during pregnancy because there are nine months when the abnormal tissue does not get a chance to grow at each cycle.

Surgery sometimes works but, because endometriosis is cell-based, it is very difficult to eliminate all growth. Hormones can be used to make the body mimic a pregnancy or menopause – so reducing the chances of the cells building up after each period. This can be done by taking contraceptive pills continuously, rather than just for your 21-day cycle, to suppress menstruation. Progesterone-based drugs may be given daily starting at a low level and then building up to a plateau which is then maintained for a further six to nine months. This also stops ovulation and the periodic shedding of the endometrium, although some women may experience breakthrough bleeding.

Danazol, derived from a synthetic male hormone, can produce a false menopause. It is taken over six to nine months but it may induce hot flushes and other symptoms of menopause.

All of these strategies may produce side effects, with progesterone causing swelling, breast tenderness, depression and other symptoms associated with pregnancy. There may be slight, temporary signs of masculinisation when using danazol because it is a male hormone derivative.

Knowing that there may be side effects, and the fact that they are temporary, helps overcome much of the anxiety.

Summing up

Experience of menstruation can differ widely among women and our perception of it is coloured by cultural and personal attitudes. It can be affected by stress, lifestyles and our general health. Make sure that, if you feel there is something that needs checking or explaining, you do not hesitate to raise the matter with your doctor. If they do not respond positively, change to another doctor.

CHAPTER FIVE

Pregnancy and Childbirth

For the first time in history women can have control over their reproductive lives. They also have a choice of contraceptive methods, though the burden is still wrongly imposed on the woman and not enough on the man. However, career women who delayed having children may find it more difficult to conceive, have a more difficult pregnancy and delivery and are also more vulnerable to conditions such as fibrocystic breasts or endometriosis. Remember that the ability to have a baby falls off naturally with age and everyone accepts that conception is more difficult after 40. But in fact it becomes more difficult in one's thirties and, in the same way, treatment of infertility is more difficult for women in their thirties.

Contraception

Too many women, young and older, still fail to ensure that precautions have been taken when they have intercourse. Unfortunately, ignorance is part of the problem, but there is also fear of the side effects of certain methods of contraception. The higher profile of the condom, because of AIDS, may help to combat some of this problem and dispel fears.

Religious and cultural restrictions limit contraception for some women but this is a matter of personal choice; they may practise abstinence, or have intercourse only during the period when they are not fertile. Birth control should be a joint effort and women should not be afraid to make that clear to their partner, particularly if it is difficult to raise because it is a casual relationship. The more they do so, the more they will help break down male taboos about this.

71

Remember, too, that the other side of the coin is planning to get pregnant. That is why care needs to be taken in the choice of IUDs, which have been known to make significant numbers of women infertile. Ask about their record. Sterilisation is also a big step that must not be entered into lightly for a woman because it is usually irreversible. This is the route that should be undertaken by men by having a vasectomy, if sterilisation is an absolute must.

Reversible contraceptives

The pill, technically known as an oral contraceptive because it is taken by mouth, remains the main birth control method for Western women. Apart from sterilisation it is also the most effective method. Doctors are still learning about the way it operates and although it seems to be safe and effective for the vast majority of women, you should make sure that you get the right one for you as an individual. Women should not go on the pill (or should come off it) if they have high blood pressure; the same goes for those who have had blood clots in their circulatory system (venous thrombosis), certain abnormalities of the liver, cancer of the breast, cervix, uterus, ovaries or other reproductive organs, or gall bladder problems. Care may need to be taken in selecting a pill for women who may have diabetes or mental depression or those who suffer from migraine. Visible signs, such as the redness around a vein in phlebitis and its associated leg pains, or high blood pressure, are indicators that you should come off the pill and check with your doctor.

The pills most in use are the combination pill and the mini-pill. The first combines synthetic forms of oestrogen and progestogen, the mini-pill containing only progestogen. The combination pill interferes with a woman's normal hormone fluctuations to prevent the egg from maturing and being released for fertilisation by the male sperm at intercourse.

Combination pills come in a variety of strengths and packaging, some containing the active 21 pills only, others with an extra seven placebo pills that have no hormone content but help you keep track of whether you have taken your pill or not during the calendar month rather than the 21-day cycle. Mini-pills have to be taken every day, so if you are forgetful you may be safer with the combination because you can normally get protection by taking two the day after you forgot.

Because women can differ so much from individual to individual, there are a range of combination pills with different amounts and types of hormone. They contain one of two types of synthetic oestrogen and one of five possible progestogens. Ringing the changes helps to cut out possible side effects such as swelling, nausea, breast tenderness and weight gain. These are associated with excess oestrogen, so a lower dosage may help, while if you get acne then more oestrogen may reduce it. In any case, it may take a few months to sort out the right pill, and acne, for example, may worsen for a month or two before clearing up.

Headaches may be caused by too much oestrogen and migraines are an indication to stop that pill. Breakthrough bleeding is most common with the mini-pill or low oestrogen formulation. Bleeding that occurs early in the cycle can usually be cleared up by adding a bit more oestrogen; late-cycle bleeding by more progestogen.

Women on the pill usually find that their periods are much lighter and free of cramps. Since ovulation stops while on the combination pill, women who suffer from PMT and/or endometriosis, may also experience relief from their symptoms. Not having a period while on the pill is normal, althogh some doctors may prescribe extra hormones once a year to bring on a period. But it is not necessary.

We explained earlier in the book that when you stop the pill it may take up to six months or longer to get back to regular menstruation and ovulation because your pill has built up a routine in your body to stop these. It is also more common when you are over 30. If it goes on for too long, some doctors prescribe a fertility drug such as clomiphene which stimulates the pituitary to produce FSH and LH.

In choosing a method of contraception, therefore, IUDs are best only for women who have completed their family. If you are young, make sure your ovaries are functioning properly and you are ovulating regularly before going on the pill. Over 30 and you will take longer to get back to normal and so possibly undermine plans to get pregnant. In either case, there is a good argument for using condoms and/or barrier methods such as spermicidal jellies during intercourse. Over 40 other side effects need to be taken into account, such as possible links to breast cancer, heart disease, and strokes. Tobacco use also comes into play as an extra risk factor.

IUDs
The spate of lawsuits in the US against manufacturers of intrauterine devices has partly been the result of the physical damage they have

caused. Laws differ from country to country, but Western women need to be very sure of their decision if they intend to use an IUD. As already said, if you plan at some stage to have a baby, then an IUD is not a good idea. It is not known how an IUD interferes with the body's normal processes to stop pregnancy, but up to six of every 100 users do become pregnant and about half of those end in miscarriage. On removal of the IUD the miscarriage rate drops to 25 per cent. But sometimes it cannot be removed safely and women who continue the pregnancy with the IUD in place have a higher risk of infection, premature delivery and stillbirth.

Many IUD pregnancies start to develop inside the fallopian tubes and are called ectopic because the embryo is developing out of place. If detected early, the tube may be saved; if the embryo continues to grow without being spotted it will rupture the tube – a serious, even life-threatening, incident for the mother. Conception for an egg from that tube may become impossible and, if the other tube is also damaged, then a woman is faced with infertility. The debate over IUDs in Europe and North America has highlighted the increase in pelvic inflammatory disease (PID), which often damages the tubes, uterus and even the ovaries. The increase has been marked amongst women with multiple sexual partners who may be exposed to a number of sexually transmitted diseases, including gonorrhoea and chlamydia, two leading causes of PID.

Barrier contraceptives
These include the diaphragm, condom, cervical cap, contraceptive sponge, contraceptive foam or jelly. Taking all factors into account, they can be the safest of all contraceptives as far one's own body is concerned and they can be used properly and consistently. Their reputation as being messy and unromantic is because they have not had the promotional support that has backed things like clotted cream cakes – messy, bad for the clothes, bad for the figure, the heart and sometimes, because of the amount of bacteria in the cream, the stomach, but nice! Apart from helping to stop AIDS transmission, barrier methods also have an important role in preventing sexually transmitted diseases.

The rhythm method
Also referred to as natural family planning, this method works by using the phase during the menstrual cycle when a woman cannot

conceive. The drawback lies in how the woman can estimate accurately when that that phase begins and ends. Not only does it demand that a woman be very aware of her body, it requires considerable checking and monitoring and there is a high failure rate. The key point is to determine when ovulation has taken place which, in theory, should be 14 days before menstruation starts. It is generally believed that sperm can live for up to four days and an egg can live for a day or two, but this may not be a good rule of thumb to follow as their lives can actually be longer, so the timing of intercourse has to be strict.

No woman has clockwork 28-day cycles month after month on which to work out a calendar-safe period. This means, therefore, that you have to work out an average of safe versus unsafe days over as long a period as possible – up to a year. Then subtract 18 days from the shortest cycle (14 days before ovulation plus four days for a sperm's life) and then calculate 11 days from the longest (14 days from ovulation until menstruation, less one day for the lifespan of an egg and two more days for a further margin of safety). This will, in theory, give you the first and last unsafe days of a woman's cycle using the first day of menstruation as day one.

So, you could have your longest cycle at 31 days and the shortest at 24. Take 11 from 31 and you get 20 days; take 18 from 24 and you get 6. You would then need to avoid intercourse from days 6 to 20 inclusive if you wished to use the rhythm method. Otherwise you could use a contraceptive.

Another way, or a possible combination, to work out when you begin ovulating, is keeping a daily record of your basal temperature. You measure it immediately on waking in the morning (before you get out of bed). This should give your lowest body temperature. The theory is that when your oestrogen and progesterone are low during the first level of the menstrual cycle your basal temperature is also low – about 97 to 97.5 degrees Fahrenheit (36.2 to 36.5 degrees Centigrade). Towards the end of the first phase of the cycle there is a slight dip in oestrogen which signals the pituitary to step up hormone production. This dip is accompanied by a corresponding drop in basal temperature. A woman keeping a temperature chart, for example, may record 97.3 degrees Fahrenheit for several days, then 96.9 and then 98, 98, 99.

The dip followed by the rise indicates that ovulation has taken place, and safe days begin about three days after that. This method is useful for determining the days that are safe after ovulation, but not in determining when intercourse should stop before ovulation takes place. One way is to assume that the unsafe period begins about six days after day one of menstruation, assuming that the woman's shortest menstrual cycle is 24 or 25 days. By and large basal temperature monitoring is not reliable, even if you can get accurate readings using electronic, automatic thermometers which use the data to calculate the 'safe period'.

There are physical signs that will tell a woman when she ovulates. One of these signs is the thickening of the mucus at the cervix until just before ovulation when it becomes thin again. Some women also experience 'mittelschmerz' – a pain which may range from a mild twinge or two to severe cramps at the time of ovulation. It is caused by bleeding when the mature egg breaks out of its follicle. But many women do not experience any pain, so it is not reliable.

One test developed for use in the home relies on monoclonal antibodies to detect the surge in luteinising hormone (LH) which occurs just before ovulation. When the LH starts to rise, ovulation should take place within 24 to 48 hours. A week or so after menstruation, you test your first morning urine with a chemically-treated stick. The test-stick changes colour if there is sufficient LH in the urine and so you know ovulation is about to take place. But these tests are probably more useful to become pregnant than to avoid it because you may have had intercourse a day or two before the test shows a rise in LH and there could be a sperm present which is still able to fertilise an egg when you do ovulate. Another US test being developed is to check the change in the cervical mucus, but progress on this and other similar tests should be asked about at specialist family planning or fertility clinics.

The morning-after pill and other postcoital methods

A French research team in mid-1989 was able to report on the use of a morning-after pill called RU486, which newspaper reports said had been tested on 30,000 women in France. Controlled trials on some 1,000 British women had also taken place. Its use in France has been accompanied by a major debate revolving around religious and ethical considerations. RU486, which temporarily blocks progesterone receptors in the womb (where they are needed to maintain a pregnancy) is combined with prostaglandin as a hormone regulator. The latter is given 48 hours later to induce complete abortion.

Obstetricians say the use of RU486 means that women would only need to spend a maximum of six hours in hospital, whereas surgical abortions mean spending one or two nights in hospital.

In the past, one method which was used and has been discontinued was to give a large dose of the synthetic oestrogen diethylstilbestrol (DES), but this has caused serious problems. If given within a day or two of unprotected intercourse DES altered the uterine lining. This prevented the egg being implanted if it had been fertilised and conception had taken place. There was concern about the side effects such as nausea, vomiting, breast tenderness and menstrual irregularities. But more much serious is that DES has been implicated in reproductive abnormalities among daughters of women who were given this synthetic oestrogen to prevent a threatened miscarriage. This use of DES was stopped in the early 1970s after reports of a rare type of vaginal cancer amongst DES daughters. Recent reports have also linked DES to an increased risk of breast cancer among women who took it years ago. Active support groups, for daughters of women who took DES, now exist in the US, France, Holland and the UK, and they are campaigning against the manufacturers. Millions of American women were known to have taken the drug. While the figures for Holland are around 100,000, in the UK there are some 8,000 women.

In the past IUDs (usually the type containing copper) have been inserted shortly after unprotected intercourse to stop a fertilised egg being implanted in the uterine wall. But bearing in mind what has been said earlier about IUDs, and also their reduced availability because a number are no longer manufactured, this is not a procedure to be undertaken lightly.

Planning a pregnancy

If you are going to have a baby then you should get in to training long before conception. The healthier you are the healthier your baby will be. If you are rundown, or have been eating badly your baby will not get the benefits it should while it is growing inside you. You should make a checklist many months before you plan starting a baby which looks at your total lifestyle: sleep, food, exercise, possible anxieties. Start thinking about reducing or cutting out tobacco, alcohol, medicines for this or that (which may only be taken because you are neglecting your health). It is also mistaken to think that only the woman has to get into training. There is plenty of evidence from the Soviet Academy of Sciences that underweight, sickly, deformed babies were the result of heavily drinking and smoking fathers.

You should prepare for a baby in the same way you would prepare for a long-distance walking holiday. Buying a cot or new boots without getting fit to use them will do no one any good! Your doctor should be brought in early so you both get a good checkup; look back through your family history for any disorders that you may need to watch for. Remember that the foetus feeds on what you feed on. If there are excessive residues of hormones in your body because you have been on the pill for a long time you need time for them to be cleared out of the body. You should take care not to use hormone-based pills by accident if you think you are pregnant. For the record, smoking (and do not forget that includes passive smoking) results in increased risks of low birthweight, miscarriages, stillbirths and possible learning problems later. Alcohol can cause small head size, facial deformities, mental retardation, heart defects, poor coordination, crossed eyes and other problems.

Narcotics should be treated in the same way as alcohol and tobacco – avoid them. You should also avoid bacteria- or virus-carrying foods which your immune system can cope with normally but threaten your growing embryo – listeria in certain dairy foods or sandwiches and pre-cooked foods from the chill cabinet, salmonella risk areas such as poorly-cooked poultry or eggs, or egg-based products such as mayonnaise. The message on food is simple – eat only the best and safest and treat your body like a brand new car which needs good oil, careful handling and no strain. Otherwise you will be building up problems for your baby when it reaches various stages through life.

If you have to take medication because of a chronic condition, then make sure you discuss it fully with your doctor and work out some kind of plan for the months before and during pregnancy. You may be able to reduce the amount or take compensatory action through your diet or lifestyle. Unnecessary X-rays should be avoided. Those signs in clinics which say 'Please tell the radiologist if you think you may be pregnant' are for real. Dental X-rays, particularly from older machines, may do no harm if you wear a lead apron, but frankly you should get all your teeth looked at long before you conceive, and bacteria released when de-scaling the teeth can affect your heart as well as that of a foetus. Antibiotics for an abscess when pregnant means the baby is getting a dose too. And in case you think it is only people who work in a chemical factory who should check out risks then think again: the lead in petrol debate may be moving behind us, but watch out for waste oil from your car and motorbike maintenance getting on your hands when you put it in the garden shed – it is highly cancerous. If you work in a photographic lab or next to a photocopier every day – check it out. Don't do DIY work which presents risks – from woodstain to loft insulation materials, from paint stripper to spraying the greenfly with insecticide. The list is long and it needs to be made and checked out in your own work and home surroundings.

If you get German measles (rubella) while you are pregnant it can cause serious birth defects in your baby. If you are not immune (check with the doctor), then you can be vaccinated three months before conceiving. The US seems to have a highly organised preventive approach that is also now developing in the UK, but practice will differ from doctor to doctor. So you may need to ask your doctor about tests, before you are eventually sent to an ante-natal clinic, when, of course, you are already pregnant. It is then normal for a variety of tests to be carried out routinely. Nowadays one blood sample can be used to carry out a whole series of tests when it goes to the hospital laboratory, and you should discuss with your doctor what you might expect. They may not, for example, think of testing for toxoplasmosis, which can seriously affect children with eye problems. It has been ignored in the past but there has been much publicity recently about the cause: infection from dog or cat faeces in parks and gardens or from household pets. If you are pregnant there's no harm in petting your cat but don't empty the cat litter box – get someone else to do it.

Becoming pregnant

When you are fit, have stopped the pill (three months before) or removed your IUD (two months before) most couples having intercourse (every two or three days) during a woman's fertile period should be able to start a pregnancy within six months. Some achieve this earlier (in the first month) and some perhaps at nine months or more. If you are getting the timing right (you can use the rhythm method calculation described earlier to work out the woman's most fertile time) and nothing happens for six months, then there is no harm in checking with your doctor. If you are 21, a delay may not be so important; if you are 35 then time matters.

Most doctors are not trained to discuss sexual technique but remember that if you are trying to help a sperm and an egg to meet, then give them time and a relaxed environment by resting after intercourse to make things easier!

Causes of infertility

Compared with marriage customs in previous centuries in Europe, far more women today either marry or have long-term relationships with a partner and have children. So there is greater awareness of infertility than in the past and more work has been done to solve it through 'test-tube' babies, a popular phrase which covers a variety of techniques to help a woman carry a baby. Because of career-delayed pregnancies there is also far more attention being given to difficulties women are having at that age when, in the past, they might have finished having children.

Taking all the age factors into account, some experts suggest that fertility problems are probably equally divided between men and women. The main cause of infertility among women is failure to ovulate and we have outlined the mechanism for this earlier in the book.

Remember how finely-balanced the hormonal system is and you will appreciate that changes in weight (through over-dieting) can stop some of the triggers working which are needed to set the chain reaction of pregnancy in motion. Increasing your weight may have a similar effect.

Disruption can occur if the pituitary does not produce enough LH and FSH to stimulate the ovaries to produce a mature egg, or the thyroid or adrenal glands may not be operating at peak efficiency.

Some women may have polycystic ovaries. This causes an imbalance in hormones:low FSH, high oestrogen, erratic surges of LH, low progesterone, raised male hormones etc. In this condition the levels of hormones tend to remain constant instead of going through the rise and fall of the menstrual cycle. The process is unclear; it is thought that a follicle swells but fails to release an egg, so it becomes a cyst. The cells around the cyst pump out weak male hormones which the body converts into oestrogen. The feedback system in the brain senses the high level of oestrogen, assumes that the ovaries are functioning properly and that a ripe egg is ready to be released. The pituitary cuts back the secretion of FSH and sends out the LH, which normally causes the ripened egg to break away from the follicle. But there is no mature egg, so the follicle forms a cyst. The high level of oestrogen prevents the uterus from being shed and this build up of the endometrium increases the risk of uterine cancer. A woman with polycystic ovaries may experience a number of other symptoms including abnormal growth of hair on the face and body and other masculine signs.

Hormonal imbalance can be the result of too much prolactin (which stimulates milk production). Stress, drugs such as the antidepressants, alcohol and painkillers as well as brain tumours and an underactive thyroid, can be the cause. It can be treated with bromocriptine, perhaps over several months, but once pregnancy occurs it should be stopped as it has been associated with birth defects.

Correcting hormonal imbalances requires a thorough analysis of the condition first, generally by an endocrinologist. About 30 per cent of women who are failing to ovulate and whose ovaries are able to produce eggs can be helped by clomiphene which tackles the lack of FSH and LH. The drug blocks the oestrogen receptors in the hypothalamus and tricks the brain into signalling the pituitary to stimulate oestrogen production by secreting FSH. This will stimulate the ovaries to ripen an egg, so producing even more oestrogen. But the hypothalamus does not sense this increase in oestrogen until the drug is stopped and then the brain detects the high levels of oestrogen and signals the pituitary to send out a surge of LH. This causes the egg to break free of the follicle, thereby completing ovulation. If the LH surge does not take place, a test for ovulation will show it up; at this stage an injection of human chorionic gonadotropin (hCG), which is similar to LH, may trigger the ovaries into releasing the ripened egg. About three-quarters of women who are not ovulating, but whose ovaries are normal, can be helped by clomiphene. Some may have twins because they may produce two eggs.

A more powerful fertility drug is made from a combination of LH and FSH obtained from the urine of menopausal women. It is collected from nuns in Italian convents and older women from Italian villages. But it acts directly on the ovaries and must be administered under very careful conditions or too many eggs could be stimulated or an ovary ruptured. It is injected during the cycle, usually from days five to 12 and regular tests are done to check the effect on the ovaries, either by measuring oestrogen levels or visually using ultrasound. The risk lies in the birth of triplets, quadruplets or more children which can be too much for the mother and so the foetuses. If it becomes evident that too many eggs are maturing the treatment should be stopped.

Mechanical causes of female infertility

In recent years there has been a growing understanding of the mechanical obstructions that can cause infertility, particularly endometriosis and blocked or damaged fallopian tubes.

Endometriosis
The cause of endometriosis and the way it prevents conception has already been discussed fully in Chapter 4. An enhanced awareness of this condition must be partly due to the fact that women are having fewer babies and at a later age than in the past. After diagnosis it usually takes six months of drug therapy to clear the disorder sufficiently to allow conception to take place. Sometimes, if the build-up of extra tissue is large or has caused scarring and distortion of the reproductive organs, surgery may also be needed, but clearing all the abnormal cells may be difficult, so the condition can return.

Tubal abnormalities
Fertilisation usually takes place in one of the fallopian tubes as the egg passes through it on its way to the uterus. But this may be prevented by blocked or scarred tubes, perhaps caused by pelvic inflammatory disease as a result of conditions such as gonorrhoea, chlamydia, or IUD use. If the embryo is caught in the tube and begins to grow there (tubal pregnancy) it can damage or destroy the tube. Microsurgery has made it possible to repair far more tubes (up to 50 per cent) than in the past, thus allowing women to begin a pregnancy.

Other causes
'Hostile' cervical mucus can prevent the sperm reaching the egg, and there are other causes such as the development of antibodies which attack the sperm, infections or conditions such as diabetes.

Causes of male infertility

Far less work has been done in this area and there are fewer treatments, although repair through microsurgery is changing the picture. Probably less than two per cent of men are completely sterile. A low sperm count is the most common cause of fertility problems. A man's sperm may in some way be defective and sperm production can be affected by alcohol or tobacco, drugs, radiation and exposure to certain chemicals and infection. Tight-fitting clothes and undergarments which constrict the scrotum and penis (as opposed to wearing, say, boxer shorts) can reduce sperm production.

Sperm are very sensitive to heat, and that is perhaps why the testes have developed outside the body to remain cooler than if they were an internal organ. Any infection or inflammation which produces even a slight rise in scrotal temperature can hinder sperm production. Not having a hot bath before intercourse is one sensible move that will increase sperm mobility. About 30 per cent of infertile men have varicocele, a condition in which a varicose vein in the testes generates heat which blocks a passageway. This can be treated either by surgery or tying it off; 70 per cent of men see improved sperm counts and half are able to fertilise a female egg after intercourse.

About 10 per cent of problems occur in the sperm transport system, perhaps a blocked or obstructed passageway. Hypospadias, where the opening of the penis is underneath instead of at the tip, makes it difficult to shoot the sperm into the vagina. Surgery for such conditions has not been very successful to date. Of course the man's sperm can be collected and introduced by other methods – artificial insemination.

Men's hormonal systems are as finely tuned as women's but hormonal causes of infertility are not as common. They should be investigated if there is no other clear cause. In a very small number of men suffering from a lack of gonadal (as with hypogonadal women) luteinizing-hormone-releasing hormone may be given; this is released periodically through a pump worn on a belt.

The pregnant body

A woman who is really attuned to her body can often tell she is pregnant before tests or seeing a doctor. Pregnancy test kits are easily available nowadays but going to see your doctor is free and his results will be more accurate – after all he is dealing with the issue every day of the week. The latest kits work by sensing the presence of hCG hormone produced by the placenta and can detect a pregnancy within two or three days of a missed period. If the test-stick shows up positive, then go and see your doctor. If it is negative and you suspect you may be pregnant, then that simply confirms the wiser course of popping along to the surgery.

The body advertises its own subtle changes when it gears up to handle a pregnancy. Almost from conception your breasts will be even more swollen and tender than usual in your immediate pre-menstrual week because of the continued rise in oestrogen and progesterone. You may experience characteristic morning sickness (it can be at any time of the day despite its name) and even vomiting at about the sixth week of pregnancy. Earlier or more pronounced morning sickness may indicate a possible multiple birth since twins in the womb cause twice as much production of oestrogen, progesterone and hCG, as one foetus.

Typically, the morning sickness continues until the 10th or 11th week and then subsides as the body adjusts to the high hormone levels. Take comfort (if you feel under the weather) from the fact that it shows your hormones are working as they should. Rarely, some women cannot keep down any food and (since you need to be thinking of your baby's intake too) you should see a doctor about ways to handle your diet. One method is to organise a number of palatable bites of bland foods through the day.

Don't be surprised if friends have no problems at all – women differ enormously and it is as normal to have morning sickness, swelling and discomfort as not to have it. If you know what to expect then the real pleasure of a baby growing inside you, and looking forward to its birth, will more than offset any trouble it puts you to in the process.

Hormonal adaptation of pregnancy

During pregnancy the thyroid gland enlarges to raise the body's metabolic rate to provide the energy needed by the foetus and the chemical changes taking place in the mother. (But do not confuse this with a rise in thyroid disease which, if it were to occur, would only happen after delivery.) Also, the parathyroid glands produce more of their hormones for calcium balance, the adrenal glands produce more aldosterone, for example, to counter sodium loss caused by high levels of progesterone, and increased cortisol helps to ensure that energy levels are sustained.

The placenta within which the foetus grows is a kind of ultimate drive-in, producing on the spot, as well as temporarily adding to the production of, hormones from organs such as the pituitary and ovaries. Despite hormone levels being increased several times than normal, a pregnant woman will not suffer any of the usual side effects that would occur if she were not pregnant. For example, the high levels of oestrogen push up angiotensin II which normally increases blood pressure – but in fact during pregnancy blood pressure is usually lower than normal!

But if a woman has toxaemia during pregnancy paradoxically there is less angiotensin II than normal, although the response to it is greater.

The stages of pregnancy

Pregnancy is divided into three periods of three months each (trimester) at 12 weeks, 27 weeks and 40 weeks. The stages of development are detailed below.

First trimester
The uterus enlarges to three times its normal size to prepare for foetal growth. The breasts also grow larger, and blood in circulation doubles (for the foetus and to compensate for loss of blood at childbirth). About 12 per cent of pregnancies end in a miscarriage, or spontaneous abortion, most occurring in this period, and usually between the sixth and 10th weeks. Ectopic (in the wrong place) pregnancies, such as those occurring in the fallopian tubes, also show up at this time. Warning signs include lower abdominal, crampy, menstrual-like pain, which may be quite severe, and vaginal spotting. It can be confirmed by blood tests, pelvic examination and ultrasound. The treatment is surgical removal of the misplaced embryo before the tube ruptures.

By week 12 the foetus weighs about 14g (half an ounce), is about 7.5cm (3in) long, has a distinctly human shape and the various organ systems are formed. You can make out its sex, ears, nose, mouth and eyes.

85

The second trimester
Most women find that this is when they bloom and glow. Morning sickness is replaced with a feeling of well-being and euphoria. While they need to wear looser clothes, the foetus is not so heavy as to make them awkward in their movements. At about week 20 you will become aware of the baby's movements, which is very exciting. By week 27 the foetus will be about 35cm (14in) long and weigh about 900g (2lb). Its movements may be so active that they wake you from a sound sleep at night.

The third trimester
The final three months of pregnancy are marked mainly by foetal growth. Kicking and movement become more pronounced and frequent; sometimes the woman will feel the baby hiccupping. There is a general feeling of awkwardness: breathing may seem more difficult and breasts become fuller and heavier. At the end of this period the baby will weigh about 3.3kg (7lb) and will be about 45–50cm (18–20in) long.

Body changes

Pregnancy and hormonal changes affect almost every part of the body and some of the more obvious that most women experience include:

Skin changes
Placental pregnancy hormone is similar to the hormone which tells the skin to produce more melanin pigment cells that give the skin its colour. Women who tan well will tan faster and deeper, so fair-skinned women can burn with only minimal exposure to the sun. Moles and freckles become darker and so do the areola around the nipples as well as becoming larger. Many women develop a dark line (linea nigra) from the navel down the abdomen to the pubic hair and this disappears a few months after delivery. Some women develop the so-called 'mask of pregnancy', dark, butterfly-shaped blotches on the face, something which may also be produced by a high oes-trogen contraceptive pill. This 'mask' sometimes disappears after delivery.

Reddish stretch marks may develop on the breasts, abdomen, and thighs and, while cream may soothe the skin, they are normal and usually fade after delivery.

Teeth and gums

Increased levels of progesterone during pregnancy expand blood supply and make gum tissue softer and spongier, so they bleed more easily. Good dental hygiene is particularly important. Massage and proper care will help maintain the gum tissue. After childbirth the swelling and bleeding will subside.

Hair

Most women notice that their hair is thicker and grows faster during pregnancy; then large amounts fall out within a few months after delivery. All hair goes through three distinct phases: a growth stage, which lasts for about three years; a resting phase of two to three months; and a shedding phase. The hormone changes of pregnancy cause a larger than usual number of hairs to go into the growing phase, and after delivery, the sharp drop in these hormones forces the hairs into the resting and shedding phases.

It is not unusual for a woman to lose up to half of her hair after a baby is born. (Interestingly, the same thing happens to the baby. Most babies are born with a lot of heavy, dark hair, which falls out shortly after birth and is replaced by fine baby hair.) Even when the mother's hair is being shed in large amounts, new hairs are growing in the shafts and within a few months, most women will again have a full head of hair. During the shedding period, a shorter, fluffier hair style will make the thinning less apparent. Avoiding hair dyes, excessive blow drying and other practices that damage hair also help, but a perm may actually 'take' better!

Vaginitis

Many women become more susceptible to vaginitis. There are several reasons for this. The hormone changes of pregnancy change the acidity of the vagina, making it more conducive to yeast and bacterial overgrowth. The increased body temperature also promotes vaginitis, as does the increased weight and more closed-in environment of the lower body as pregnancy progresses.

Bowel and urinary changes

Pregnant women often feel that their entire waste-disposal mechanism has gone awry, and to a degree, they are right. The hormonal changes relax the smooth muscles, including those of the intestines, and this can lead to diarrhoea, constipation or a combination of the two. The increased pressure of the expanding uterus affects both the bladder and colon. During pregnancy, women find they need to unrinate more frequently, and some may have problems with involuntary loss of small amounts of urine. This is caused by the bladder being pushed out of its normal position, and also by the muscle relaxation that accompanies the hormone changes. The pregnant woman also has an increased blood volume and a change in fluid balance, which often results in fluid retention and swelling.

Swollen hands and feet
Toward the end of pregnancy, most women experience mild oedema or swelling of the hands and feet. This is caused by increased fluid retention due to the expanded blood supply, pressure of the expanding uterus, and a tendency for blood to 'pool', or collect, in the lower part of the body. It is not a cause for worry unless the swelling is accompanied by headaches, high blood pressure and other symptoms, in which case the doctor should be called immediately. Diuretics (water pills) should be avoided unless specifically recommended by a doctor. Instead one should try cutting down on salt, sitting with the feet resting on a stool and lying down with legs up a couple of times a day. Tight knee-high socks should be avoided. Wearing a larger size shoe also eases foot discomfort – a rather obvious solution, but one that a suprising number of women overlook.

Allergy and sinus congestion
Hay fever and other allergies sometimes become worse during pregnancy, and many women find that they also are more susceptible to sinus congestion, postnasal drip and sinus headaches. The hormonal changes of pregnancy cause a swelling of the nasal tissues; this, combined with the increased venous pressure, results in increased production of nasal secretions. Saline nose drops may help, as may a cold-water humidifier that moistens room air. Increased headaches, especially tension headaches related to the back discomfort that is common during the latter part of pregnancy, may also be troubling. Massage and relaxation exercises often help. Acetaminophen may be acceptable as a pain reliever; it is not as likely to cause bleeding problems as aspirin. All medications, including over-the-counter drugs, should be checked with a doctor before use.

Varicose veins and haemorrhoids

Many pregnant women are troubled by varicose veins and haemor-rhoids (which are varicose veins in the anus). These are caused by the increased abdominal weight and pressure, the larger blood volume of pregnancy and the effect of progesterone, which relaxes the muscle wall in the veins. They usually disappear after childbirth, and can be minimised by common-sense measures. Resting with the legs elevated, wearing elastic stockings, avoiding prolonged periods of standing or sitting with the legs in the same position and exercise can all relieve or lighten the discomfort. Haemorrhoids can be relieved by increasing the amount of roughage in the diet to help prevent consti-pation, and avoiding straining during a bowel movement.

Leg cramps

Caused by fluxes in the body's electrolyte balance, leg cramps often happen at night. They occur when fluxes of sodium, calcium and po-tassium atoms increase. Blood levels of these substances do not neces-sarily reflect their activity in the leg muscles; thus, increasing the oral intake of calcium, as is sometimes suggested, may not ease the cramping. A better approach is to do stretching exercises to relax the leg muscles and make them less prone to cramping.

Feelings of euphoria, fatigue and insomnia

Many women experience euphoria during pregnancy, partly due to the increase in steroids. The euphoria all too often turns to de-pression following the baby's birth, due to the sharp decrease in oes-trogen after delivery. Fortunately, the depression is usually temporary.

Many women experience bursts of energy at different times, interspersed with marked feelings of fatigue. This is often com-pounded by insomnia, especially towards the end. There are numerous explanations for these feelings. During the foetal growth spurts and near the end of pregnancy, a woman uses a tremendous amount of energy simply providing for the fast-growing baby. She needs to rest more often, and an afternoon nap may well become ne-cessary to get through to an early bedtime. At the same time, many pregnant women are troubled by insomnia. It may be difficult for them to find a comfortable sleeping position, and they no sooner fall asleep than they are wakened by the need to go to the toilet, or by leg cramp or the baby suddenly kicking and turning. Some women find it helpful to take a walk before going to bed or do relaxation exercises. Sleeping with extra pillows may make breathing easier. In any event, sleeping pills should be avoided, since these are among the drugs that can cause birth defects.

As full term approaches and the baby 'drops', most women find they can again breathe normally because the foetus is no longer pressing against the lungs. You may experience a renewed burst of energy before the onset of labour. Accounts of labour beginning while undertaking tasks unthinkable a few weeks earlier – scrubbing the kitchen floor or re-tiling a bathroom – are common.

Heartburn
Indigestion is common and during the early stages may be related to morning sickness, later to increased abdominal pressure on the stomach. This causes a backup of gases and gastric juices into the oesophagus. The problem practically always disappears a day or two after delivery. Eating frequent, small meals and avoiding food that cause gassiness and acid secretion usually helps. Foods which aggravate heartburn are coffee, tea, orange juice and piquant spices. A doctor's advice should be sought before taking antacids. Sodium bicarbonate, which increases fluid retention and can cause a rise in blood pressure, should be avoided.

What the doctor looks for during pregnancy

Regular check-ups are essential during the course of a pregnancy. A woman should know what the ante-natal clinic staff is checking for and why, and be aware of any warning signs herself that may signal a developing problem. Some of these are obvious, such as vaginal spotting or bleeding, which may signal a miscarriage. Premature contractions are normal and common in late pregnancy but they may indicate the onset of early labour. Other signs are more subtle and need to be checked for by the doctor. These include:

Abnormal weight gain
This may be due to abnormal fluid retention, which may be a sign of developing toxaemia. On the other hand, if a woman does not gain weight as she is suppposed to, there may be something wrong with the pregnancy.

90

Blood pressure
If this is on the high side your doctor or nurse may check it each day for perhaps a week. Rising blood pressure may be a warning sign of toxaemia, and needs to be carefully watched because of the dangers it can cause both mother and baby. It is normal for blood pressure to drop by the second trimester. This may cause dizziness when standing too long. Normal pressure during pregnancy is less than 120/80mm hg. As more women are becoming pregnant at a later age, elevation of blood pressure has become more common, because high blood pressure is more common as aging occurs. A pregnant woman over the age of 35 probably should have her blood pressure checked every two weeks until her third trimester, and weekly thereafter.

Elevated blood sugar and sugar in the urine
These are warning signs of gestational diabetes, a leading cause of stillbirths and early neonatal deaths. It is vital that gestational diabetes be detected early in pregnancy, and steps taken to normalise the mother's blood sugar.

Foetal heartbeat
The baby's heartbeat is checked on every visit. A doctor should also do periodic pelvic examinations.

Tests that may be performed

There are some tests that doctors may recommend to be absolutely sure that all is going well with mother and baby. These include:

Ultrasound
Waves of sound are picked up by a microphone to map internal struc- tures. Ultrasound is useful in determining whether the baby is devel- oping normally and whether there is more than one foetus. Ultra- sound does not expose the baby to radiation and is considered safe, although the long-term effects of sound waves are unknown and under debate.

Amniocentesis
This test involves withdrawing a small amount of the amniotic fluid surrounding the foetus and analysing it for signs of genetic or chro- mosomal defects. It is done most frequently in older women (over 35)

who have an increased risk of having a baby with Down's syndrome, a chromosomal abnormality. The fluid can also be used to detect Tay Sachs disease and certain other hereditary disorders, but these analyses are not done unless there is reason to believe that the baby may be at risk. A newer, still experimental, test involves suctioning out a sample of cells shed by the foetus very early in pregnancy and analysing them for defects. This test, called chorionic villus sampling, carries a somewhat higher risk of causing a miscarriage than amniocentesis, but has the advantage of detecting possible problems earlier in a pregnancy when an abortion is easier to do.

Complications of pregnancy

Most women experience an uncomplicated, albeit exciting pregnancy followed by normal delivery. But, now and then, complications do develop. Increasingly, these can be spotted early and successfully treated. There are however, inevitable pregnancy losses, often due to gross abnormalities in the foetus. In this sense, a miscarriage is a blessing in disguise, but still a painful experience for the couple. Some of the more common complications of pregnancy include:

Gestational diabetes
This disorder occurs in perhaps up to 5 per cent of all pregnancies, making it the most common medical complication of pregnancy. In some countries the incidence may be higher. In Mexico, for example, gestational diabetes occurs in more than 10 per cent of all pregnancies.

As its name implies, gestational diabetes is high blood sugar that occurs during pregnancy, and then disappears as soon as the baby is born. It is a result of a genetic predisposition to diabetes and the stress of pregnancy.

Even under normal circumstances, pregnancy demands increased insulin production, because of the increased metabolic activity. Oestrogen, progesterone and human placental lactogen are somewhat anti-insulin in nature, and so the need for more cortisol arises during pregnancy, and exerts a marked effect on glucose metabolism by increasing the conversion of glycogen stored in the liver to glucose. Women with a tendency to diabetes may not be able to handle all these extra demands, and will develop gestational diabetes, usually without any warning or symptoms. The onset is usually during the second trimester. Since the mother's blood sugar levels usually are not high enough to produce the characteristic symptoms of diabetes – excessive thirst and urination, hunger and weight loss – it can go undetected unless the doctor tests for it.

Failure to detect and treat it can cause the foetus to produce insulin prematurely, and to store the extra sugar as fat. As a result of this constant overnutrition these babies are abnormally large at birth – often weighing about 4kg (9lb) or more.

Because of the extra insulin in its blood, the baby often cannot stabilise its own blood glucose levels after birth, and may sufffer sudden life-threatening drops in blood glucose. Gestational diabetes is the major cause of stillbirths and a leading cause of death or serious illness of newborn babies. Women with it also frequently have problems later and about half will get Type 2 diabetes as they age (see Chapter 10).

So all pregnant women should be tested at some point between the 24th and 28th weeks of pregnancy, usually two hours after a meal and also when fasting. A special diet is used to normalise blood sugar, plus insulin if necessary. Several injections of insulin each day may be required and the woman must learn how to match her insulin dosage to her food intake and exercise. To ensure that she maintains a normal blood sugar level at all times, she will probably also be taught a simple home test to measure her own blood glucose.

Women who have had gestational diabetes in one pregnancy are likely to develop it in subsequent pregnancies. Not infrequently, undiagnosed gestational diabetes is responsible for a poor obstetrical history – habitual miscarriages, stillbirths, toxaemia, large, sick babies or recurrent urinary tract infections. A woman at high risk of diabetes – i.e. with a family history of the disease, obesity, gestational diabetes in a previous pregnancy, poor pregnancy outcomes, or birthweights more than about 4kg (9lb) – should be tested for gestational diabetes several times during pregnancy.

Hypertension

High blood pressure is an age-old complication of pregnancy. If a woman has high blood pressure before pregnancy, she should talk to her doctor about any medication she is taking and the special risks she may encounter in trying to have a baby. Increasingly, women with hypertension are having normal pregnancies, but the babies are apt to be smaller than usual because the blood supply to the foetus is somewhat less than normal. Complications such as a partially-detached placenta (placental abruption), and toxaemia, are more common among women with hypertension.

Dizziness and fainting

Dizziness or feeling faint, especially during the third trimester, is caused by a pooling of blood in the legs, and also by lowered pressure. Women should avoid getting out of bed too quickly, or standing up abruptly after bending over or sitting down.

Urinary tract infections

Women who are prone to cystitis or kidney infections are especially susceptible to them during pregnancy. The expanding uterus puts extra pressure on the bladder, and may impede the flow of urine. Sometimes a developing urinary infection may go unnoticed because pregnant women experience an increased need to urinate. But any burning, blood in the urine or other signs of infection should be checked promptly by a doctor, and treated with the approporiate antibiotic. Some antibiotics, such as tetracycline and sulpha drugs, should not be taken during pregnancy, but there are safe alternatives. Letting the infection go untreated poses a threat to both mother and baby.

Herpes

Some women have the mistaken idea that herpes inevitably means problems for the baby, or at least, that she must have the baby by Caesarean section. This is not the case, although a woman with genital herpes does need to exercise certain precautions. A Caesarean is necessary only if she shows signs of an active herpes virus near the time of delivery. The doctor should check her frequently during the last month of pregnancy and if there is an active flare-up, then vaginal delivery may be too risky for the baby and a Caesarean may be performed. Otherwise women with herpes can experience normal vaginal deliveries.

Placenta previa

In this disorder, the placenta is implanted low in the uterus and covers part or all of the cervical opening. As pregnancy progresses and the cervix begins to thin out and dilate, the placental attachment to the uterus is disturbed and bleeding may occur. In some women, this is mild and the pregnancy proceeds without undue problems. In others, however, the bleeding may be profuse and require hospitalisation and transfusions and, if the placenta covers all or most of the cervix, a Caesarean delivery.

Premature labour

Prematurity is the major cause of death and serious disability in the newborn. Although tremendous advances have been made in treating and saving premature babies some are left with life-long physical and mental handicaps. Thus a major goal of pregnancy is to deliver the baby at term – either too early or too late can be detrimental.

Sometimes prematurity is caused by a weak, or incompetent cervix. In this condition, the cervix is abnormally dilated and, when the foetus reaches a certain size (usually in the second trimester), a miscarriage takes place. This can be prevented by sewing the cervix to close it early in the pregnancy; the stitches are removed with the onset of labour for a normal delivery.

The causes of premature labour are poorly understood, mainly because it is not known precisely what initiates labour, even at term. It happens in about 5 per cent of all pregnancies. Of course, the risk for the baby depends upon how premature labour is. Of the babies born after 28 weeks of gestation, by which time they weigh slightly less than 900g (about 2lb), about half survive, provided they get intensive care. If the baby weighs 1.3kg (3lb), the chances of survival rise to 90 per cent.

The first sign of premature labour is usually uterine contractions. Sometimes there is vaginal bleeding or an increase in vaginal discharge. In about 20 to 30 per cent of cases, there is a premature rupture of the amniotic sac.

If at all possible, steps should be taken to halt premature contractions unless the pregnancy is close enough to term to ensure that the baby's lungs are sufficiently developed to sustain normal breathing. The woman should contact her doctor immediately. Bed rest, sometimes for the remainder of the pregnancy, is mandatory. In addition, there are several ways of halting the contractions.

The drug ritodrine can stop them, and if the woman appears stable she may be sent home to continue taking the drug in pill form. Its action is unclear and some women do not like it because it sends up their pulse rate. Although it has lowered the mortality rate from prematurity, its use is limited and it is not necessarily appropriate for women with heart disease or certain other conditions including toxaemia, uncontrolled high blood pressure, or asthma that may be being treated with a similar drug or with steroids. Ritodrine causes a rise in blood sugar; thus, if it is necessary to use this drug in a diabetic woman, the insulin doses need to be increased, sometimes even doubled. In addition, ritodrine causes a drop in potassium levels. Other possible side effects include increased pulse rate, palpitations, feelings of nervousness, nausea and vomiting, tremor and a skin rash. Although unpleasant, the side effects usually can be tolerated, especially with the knowledge that they are temporary and the baby's chances for survival are improving the longer the pregnancy can continue. Terbutaline is a drug similar to ritodrine, and another possible choice is the anti-spasmodic salbutamol which is also used by asthmatics.

Alcohol will also relax the uterus, and taking a stiff drink of whisky, gin or some other alcoholic beverage every few hours may be recommended for women experiencing premature contractions. Some women question this strategy since they have been cautioned not to drink alcoholic beverages during a pregnancy because of the possibility of causing congenital abnormalities. Since the baby is fully formed, this amount of alcohol will not cause birth defects. Premature labour is an instance in which the benefits of the use of alcohol outweigh the possible hazards to the foetus.

Labour and delivery

Labour can be induced by giving a woman an infusion of the hormone oxytocin at or near term. At one time it was thought that this hormone, which is produced by the pituitary gland, initiated labour, but further studies have indicated that it acts more as a messenger to promote the progression of labour rather than the one that actually starts it.

Animal studies seem to indicate that the signal that triggers labour may come from the foetus itself. This has led to the theory that when the foetal brain, pituitary and adrenal glands reach a certain stage of maturity, they produce hormones that are secreted into the foetal membranes. This causes increased production of prostaglandins, which in turn soften the cervix and cause uterine contractions in the mother.

While this theory may hold for some animal species, it is not clear that it applies to humans. Prostaglandins clearly play a key role in

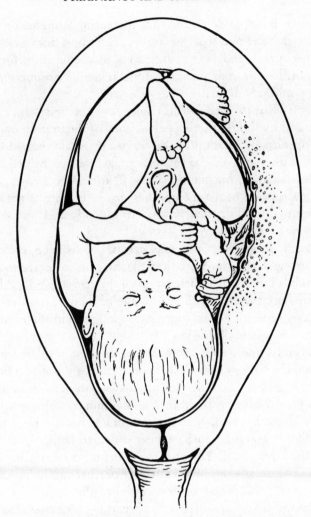

*Figure 10. The foetus at full term: the drawing shows the foetus
at 22.5 per cent of actual size*

labour, but what prompts their increased production, is unknown,
though it may be increased oestrogen and lowered progesterone.
Perhaps the excessive stretching of the uterus and foetal membranes,
as pregnancy reaches term, results in increased prostaglandins. Before
the actual onset of labour, women experience painless contractions of
the uterus. These are called Braxton-Hicks contractions, and are
sometimes confused with the onset of labour. They produce a hardening of the uterus, similar to that which occurs during labour

contractions, but they do not become increasingly intense or frequent or change the character of the cervix. Braxton-Hicks contractions 'prime' the uterus and soften the cervix in preparation for labour. These contractions may increase prostaglandin production in the uterus and initiate labour.

Labour itself is divided into three stages. The first stage, which is characterised by the rhythmic contractions of the uterine muscle and gradual opening or dilation of the cervix, is usually heralded by the 'show', the discharge of the mucous plug that has helped hold the cervix closed during pregnancy. There also may be a rush of water, signalling a rupture of the membranes. In the beginning the contractions are usually mild; they last 10–20 seconds and may be 20–30 minutes apart.

As labour progresses and the cervix opens, the contractions become stronger and more frequent, lasting up to 50 seconds. They may be only a minute or two apart, until the cervix is fully dilated, or open, signalling the end of the first stage of labour. In all, this stage usually lasts 12 to 14 hours, but may be longer with first babies and shorter in subsequent deliveries.

The second stage begins after the cervix is fully dilated and continues until the baby is born. The contractions are not as painful and the woman gets a 'second wind'. This is fortunate because now, after hours of enduring painful, but involuntary muscle work, the woman is asked to work with her voluntary muscles until the baby is born. She is asked to push or bear down to help move the baby through the birth canal. The pushing effort must be timed with contractions. The doctor, midwife, nurse or partner can help, telling her when to push and when to rest and breathe deeply in between pushes. In the first stage of labour, breathing exercises are used to lessen the perception of pain; in the second stage, the woman needs to breathe deeply to fill her lungs for the period when she is pushing and not breathing.

By this time, many women are tired and find it difficult to push as instructed. It's a poor time to try to be a good student. A woman should go to ante-natal classes that teach her how to cope with labour; then having her partner on hand to help her through labour and delivery will be a great support.

An episiotomy, an incision that usually goes from the vagina toward the rectum, may need be done to prevent tearing of the skin and shorten the second stage of labour. But ask about this in advance; research shows too many have been done unnecessarily.

In the normal birth sequence, the baby's head emerges first, preferably facing downward. After the head has emerged, it is turned sideways, and the shoulders and the rest of the body quickly follow. The umbilical cord, which attaches the baby to the placenta, is clamped and cut. The baby usually takes a breath and begins to cry loudly on its own; sometimes a small catheter will be needed to gently suction the baby's nose and mouth to permit it to breathe. Within the first minute or so, the baby will be carefully checked to make sure that it is breathing properly and everything is normal. It may then be passed to the mother or placed in a bassinet.

The third and final stage of labour entails the delivery of the afterbirth, or placenta. This usually happens within a few minutes of birth; if not, the doctor may have to remove it. If an episiotomy was done, it will be stitched shut. The woman also may be given a shot of the hormone oxytocin to stimulate further uterine contractions and help stop any bleeding.

Special considerations

In the last decade, there has been increased emphasis on so-called natural childbirth, a term that has come to describe delivery without anaesthesia, forceps or other aids. Obviously, childbirth is a natural event, and there is some merit in arguments that a delivery free of anaesthesia, forceps or a vacuum extractor may be safer for the baby. But there are instances in which these aids are needed, and a woman should not feel that she has somehow 'failed' because she needed a painkiller or that the baby needed extra help in being born.

Foetal monitoring
Early in labour, an external foetal monitor may be attached and will remain in place until the baby is born. The monitor is a microphone which picks up the baby's heart rate and measures uterine contractions. It can show a sudden drop in the baby's heart rate – a sign that the baby may be in trouble and that delivery should take place immediately.

Some advocates of 'natural' childbirth object to foetal monitoring. In reality, the monitor does not interfere with normal labour and delivery. The mother is hardly aware of the monitor and it can offer added protection for the foetus in case something goes wrong.

However, indications are that foetal monitoring leads doctors, particularly younger, inexperienced ones, to intervene unnecessarily because the monitoring equipment is throwing out unusual or unfamiliar signals. In the USA this is compounded by fear of lawsuits; insurance rates for obstetricians have risen significantly in countries like the UK for the same reason.

Caesarean section

Research has shown that Caesarean rates have gone up significantly in the US; in the UK they made up 15 per cent of all deliveries in the mid-Eighties. This is a high figure compared to countries like Holland (around 5 per cent). An obstetrician's attitude towards Caesareans should be discussed beforehand – you may need to check with the midwife to find out a hospital's practice. Midwives in general aim to do all they can to help a woman have her delivery with minimum intervention.

Most Caesarean sections are unplanned and are performed at the last minute – because the baby or mother are in distress or some other problem develops that makes surgical delivery safer. In other instances, a Caesarean may be planned almost from the outset of pregnancy because it is clear that a vaginal delivery will be unsafe. Increasingly Caesarean sections are done with a local anaesthetic (an epidural block) so the mother can be awake for the delivery of her baby. Some hospitals also permit the father in the operating room during a Caesarean.

If a woman has one Caesarean, that all her subsequent babies must be born by Caesarean is not necessarily true. Depending upon the type of incision on the uterus and the reason for the first Caesarean, it is possible that future babies may be delivered vaginally. A pregnant woman should ask for a copy of her hospital record (if a previous delivery was by Caesarean); this will indicate what type of incision she has had on her uterus, so her doctor can determine if a future vaginal delivery is feasible. The scar on the abdomen does not necessarily reflect what type of incision was used on the uterus. A horizontal incision on the lower part of the uterus is less likely to rupture during a subsequent labour than the classic vertical one. Women who have this type of Caesarean incision may be able to have a safe vaginal delivery, provided that the reasons for the first Caesarean no longer apply.

In considering the possibilities of a Caesarean, it is important to realise that 95 per cent of the time everything goes as planned and a woman can have a normal vaginal delivery. In 3 to 5 per cent of cases, however, there are problems in which a Caesarean is a better choice. Undoubtedly, some of these women would be able to deliver their babies if labour were allowed to proceed, while others would encounter major, even life-threatening problems. Although a Caesarean is disappointing to a couple that have planned a vaginal delivery (it also entails longer recuperation and a greater risk of complications for the mother) not many doctors or parents want to take any chance that may be a risk to the baby.

Induced labour

Artificial induction of labour is not as common today as in the past. Again the incidence has been high in the UK and higher in different regions, for no good reason. The same applies to episiotomies. But there are times when labour should be induced. For example, if a woman goes a week beyond her due date and there is no sign of labour, it may be induced. Just as it is in the best interest of the foetus not to be born too soon, it also is preferable not to let the baby go more than a few days beyond the due date. As pregnancy reaches its full term, the placenta begins to age, and the baby may not get adequate nutrition.

Some US obstetricians may advise sexual intercourse as pregnancy nears term because the prostaglandins in the seminal fluid may help soften the cervix and promote uterine contractions. In the past, couples often were advised to avoid sex during the last part of pregnancy because of fears of infections. We now know that sex does not lead to infection, unless, of course, the membranes have been ruptured or the man has an infection that can be sexually transmitted. Sex also should be avoided if the woman is threatening premature labour.

If indicated, labour can be induced by administering oxytocin, provided that pregnancy is full-term. Sometimes a gel containing prostaglandins may be inserted into the vagina to soften the cervix before giving oxytocin. An injection of oxytocin may also be given if labour seems to be slowing down or stalling. Labour that goes on and on, but is not producing increased dilation of the cervix can pose serious problems for the baby. This is acceptable if the contractions are producing progressive labour, but if they are not and are allowed to go on too long, the baby may experience too much oxygen deprivation.

If a woman who has had a previous Caesarean section, and is now planning a vaginal delivery, goes beyond her due date, she may have to have another Caesarean, even if all else appears normal. It is not safe to induce labour with oxytocin in this situation because it produces very strong uterine contractions and raises the risk of rupture of the uterus at the old scar site.

Hormonal changes following delivery

During pregnancy, the placenta has served as a hormone-making factory, modifying the role of the ovaries and pituitary. Before her normal hormonal function returns, a woman may experience many of the symptoms commonly associated with menopause: irritability, mood swings and depression.

Many women and their husbands are bewildered by these symptoms, especially the post-partum depression. A woman has experienced nine months of joyful anticipation of having a baby; now that the baby is here the mother finds herself bursting into tears or feeling sad for no apparent reason. If she understands that these feelings have a hormonal rather than psychological basis, she may find it easier to cope. In rare instances, the depression becomes so severe that it requires treatment. Traditionally, doctors treat this severe post-partum depression with powerful drugs, such as chlorpromazine, but a sympathetic psychiatrist, with experience of post-partum depression problems would be the best person to consult.

Fortunately, in most instances, the non-pregnant body adjusts to its new hormone state in a few days and the post-partum blues and other such symptoms subside to a more manageable state. But the body will require several months to resume its pre-pregnancy functions. It usually takes several weeks for the uterus to heal fully and for post-delivery bleeding to stop.

Menstruation usually resumes in three or four months, but if a woman breastfeeds, the high levels of prolactin needed to make breastmilk act to suppress ovulation, so a woman may not have her period for six months. Undoubtedly, ancient wise men took note of this fact and, in some societies, women nurse their babies far longer than is necessary as a means of birth control. Among some African societies, for example, a woman may nurse for three or more years and, during this time, she and her baby live apart from her husband, who may have more than one wife.

Bones and ligaments may require several months to regain their pre-pregnancy strength. For this reason, doctors advise that women use caution in resuming vigorous exercise programmes. Toning exercises, such as modified sit-ups, leg-lifts and yoga exercises to improve bladder control and tone the vaginal muscles can start shortly after childbirth. But vigorous exercises, such as jogging, should be approached cautiously. All women are different, however, and this is an instance in which a woman should take cues from her body. If exercise hurts, it's an indication to ease up and work up gradually.

Many women are distressed to find that when they come home from the hospital they still have to wear maternity clothes. It often takes several months for a woman to regain her trim pre-pregnancy figure. Toning exercises to strengthen abdominal muscles will help, but a flat stomach doesn't return overnight.

Weight gained during pregnancy also may be difficult to shed, especially if a woman breastfeeds. On average a woman can expect to very quickly lose 9kg (20lb) following delivery, since this is the normal weight gain to support the pregnancy plus the weight of the baby. So, 4kg (9lb) for the baby, placenta and membranes; about 1kg (2lb) of amniotic fluid; 1.6 kg (3½lb) for extra fluid; 500g (1lb) in breast enlargement; 1kg (2lb) in the enlarged uterus; and about 1kg (2lb) of extra body fluid. But the average recommended weight gain during pregnancy is 11-14kg (25-30lb), so many women find they have some extra weight to shed if they want to achieve their pre-pregnancy weight, as they usually do.

Women who breastfeed find this particularly hard to do, for several reasons. The hunger centre in the brain responds to the body's need for extra food to feed the baby by sending out stronger messages. As a result, most women find they have a ravenous appetite during breastfeeding, and that it takes almost superhuman will power to reduce food intake at this time. Since breastfeeding should be a happy time for both mother and baby, it may be a good idea to postpone trying to lose extra weight until after the baby is weaned.

Menstruation usually resumes in three to six months, although it may take a month or two longer for women who breastfeed. The most common cause for failure to resume menstruation is another pregnancy; many women mistakenly think that if they breastfeed or have not yet had a period, they are safe from getting pregnant. This is not necessarily true, and if a woman wants to avoid pregnancy, she should practice birth control as soon as she resumes sexual relations.

Sometimes pituitary dysfunction is the cause of a woman's failure to resume menstruation. It may be necessary to 'wake up' the pituitary and re-start normal menstrual cycles. The first stage is to determine the degree of lack of pituitary function. Clomiphene may be prescribed to gauge the pituitary response. But in some cases there may not be a response and there may be a deficiency of other pituitary trophic hormones. This must be treated by appropriate hormones. Oestrogen replacement may follow to get the ovaries working again. After ovulation takes place, the monthly cycles should resume.

Practical pointers

Almost from the moment of its birth, a woman establishes a very special bonding with her baby. Recent studies confirm the importance of letting the mother hold and react with her newborn infant immediately after delivery. In instances where this is not possible – for example, cases in which the baby requires special treatment in a neonatal unit – other steps should be taken to let the mother hold or help care for the baby.

A number of other important decisions need to be made, either before or just after the baby is born. These include whether or not to breastfeed. Although modern formulas provide adequate nutrition, breastfeeding, even if only for a short time, is superior and provides important immunity from infection for the baby. Almost all women are capable of breastfeeding, but there may be circumstances that prevent it, or a woman may simply choose not to nurse. Women who do not want to breastfeed, or who are trying to wean a baby, should avoid breast stimulation for a few days.

Summing up

Pregnancy is a major milestone in any woman's life. It is also a time when her entire endocrine system undergoes profound change geared towards producing a healthy baby. Knowing what to expect and heeding the warning signs of possible problems will make sure that all does go well.

CHAPTER SIX

Menopause

Menopause is a word that many of us don't even like to utter. Women anticipate it with apprehension. Both sexes mistakenly regard it as a sign that a woman is 'over the hill'. Fortunately, these attitudes are changing as an increasing number of women in their fifties and beyond are demonstrating that they can hold their own in the boardroom and the bedroom; indeed many of the world's most influential and glamorous women are 50 and older.

Popularly referred to as 'the change', menopause is when ovulation and menstruation cease, thus marking the end of a woman's reproductive years. Menopause is also referred to as the female climacteric, meaning 'top rung of the ladder'. It has more of a psychosocial connotation than a clinical one, and highlights the fact that menopause is both a biological and a sociological/emotional event, and it is often difficult to separate the two.

Today, the average age of menopause is about 51, and a woman's expected life span has advanced to 78. So, when a woman enters menopause in the 1990s, she can anticipate that a third of her life still lies ahead.

This does not negate the fact that a woman does encounter change with menopause, and that these changes often bring troublesome symptoms and physical and emotional problems. Still, new insight and understanding can minimise the symptoms and emotional trauma.

Menopause is a gradual process that covers five to 10 years, during which the ovarian function slows down and then stops completely. At birth, a baby girl has about two million follicles, or egg-forming cells, in her ovaries and the number drops to 500,000 by puberty. From then on, one or two of these follicles will mature, or ripen, during each menstrual cycle, and others will die. As a woman approaches menopause, she will have only about 8,000 remaining follicles. Even though the pituitary produces more follicle-stimulating hormone with each cycle, ovulation does not always take place. Low oestrogen levels result in a change in the nature of the menstrual period.

There are three stages. The first is pre-menopause, during which the ovaries gradually decrease in their function. Periods become irregular and more infrequent, but some women find they may have two periods two or three weeks apart, then go six or eight weeks without one.

The menstrual flow itself changes. Most women notice that their periods are lighter and more watery, with less clot-like substances. Others find they have a very heavy flow for one or two days, then several days of thin spotting. (Several days of spotting before menstruation may also be a sign of pre-menopause.) Still other women will have very heavy bleeding.

In the second stage, ovarian function declines further and periods stop completely. After a woman has gone a full year without menstruating, menopause is complete and she enters the post-menopausal stage of life. The term 'perimenopausal' is used to describe all three stages.

The age at which menopause happens varies widely. Some women begin in their early 40s, others not until their mid-50s.

Symptoms associated with menopause

Menopause varies from woman to woman. Some are barely aware of it until they suddenly realise that several months have passed since their last menstrual period. At the other extreme, some women suffer from frequent, almost incapacitating hot flushes, night sweats, depression, mood swings, irritability, insomnia and other symptoms which may continue for several years. Most women fall somewhere in between, but all women experience a marked change in hormonal status.

Menopause may be accompanied by a wide range of symptoms, most related to hormonal changes. As the ovaries cease to function, they no longer produce oestrogen. In response, the pituitary sends out

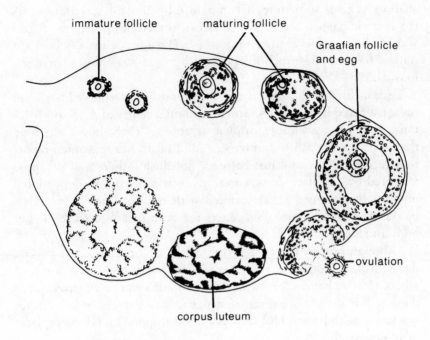

immature follicle   maturing follicle

Graafian follicle
and egg

ovulation

corpus luteum

Figure 11.   Development of ovarian follicles

more luteinising hormone (LH) and follicle-stimulating hormone (FSH) in a futile attempt to stimulate the ovaries into action.

Often, irregular or skipped periods are the first signs of menopause. Not uncommonly, a woman who misses one or two periods and has no other symptoms may think she is pregnant and use an at-home urine test. These tests are more likely to give a false positive result in women approaching menopause than in younger women, so further testing is needed before making the assumption that pregnancy is the reason for the lack of menstruation.

Although menopausal symptoms are frequently attributed to a lack of oestrogen, in some women oestrogen plays an indirect role, with the symptoms actually due to the high levels of LH or FSH.

Hot flushes
Three out of four women experience hot flushes. During a hot flush a woman experiences a sudden rush of heat to her upper body, starting in the chest area and rapidly spreading to the face, neck and arms.

The skin reddens, her heart beats faster and breathing becomes more shallow. This is sometimes accompanied by an itching sensation. As the episode passes, she begins to sweat, sometimes profusely. Afterwards, she may feel chilly and drained. The episode usually lasts for only a few minutes and others with her may not notice anything unusual.

Technically hot flushes are called vasomotor instability. They seem to be triggered by the temperature-regulating centre of the hypothalamus, and, for susceptible women, it appears that almost anything that affects temperature can trigger a hot flush. Many women report they feel a sudden chill just before a hot flush; others find it can be triggered by exercise, stress, entering a warm or cool room, or lying under a blanket in bed. Associated with the hot flush is increased blood flow in the skin. This causes the rush of blood to the upper body and face.

Although hot flushes result from a lack of oestrogen, the precise mechanism is unknown. However, women born without ovaries, or whose ovaries have never functioned, do not seem to experience hot flushes. But if they are given oestrogen, they may have hot flushes when it is withdrawn. Hot flushes can be stopped by taking replacement oestrogen.

Some women never experience hot flushes at all, while others may have several each day or even every hour. Others may experience them only at night. Night sweats are similar to those that may occur following childbirth – a time of abrupt hormonal change. You many wake up in a drenching sweat several times a night, and this may be a factor in insomnia experienced during menopause.

For many, hot flushes end in three to five years. But for some they last for only a few months, while others may have them for five or more years. Sometimes they end and then reappear years later. (Interestingly, older men also may experience hot flushes.)

Although hot flushes can be halted by taking oestrogen, there are some women for whom hormone replacement therapy is contra-indicated or who would prefer not to use it. The symptoms may be minimised by such commonsense measures as wearing several layers of light clothing so some can be shed if the need arises, and, if possible, taking a tepid shower. Caffeine and alcohol seem to aggravate the symptoms in some women and should be avoided if they trigger hot flushes. Some drugs, such as those used to treat high blood pressure, may also aggravate the vasomotor instability.

If so, an alternative may be prescribed. Large doses of niacin, or nicotinic acid – a B vitamin that some people take in large amounts to lower cholesterol – also precipitate hot flushes. (In fact, men on high doses of niacin often say, after having a few hot flushes themselves, that they suddenly understand why women are troubled by them.)

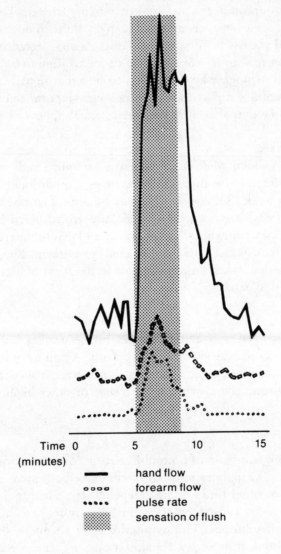

Time 0   5   10   15
(minutes)

——— hand flow
○○○○ forearm flow
••••• pulse rate
░░░░ sensation of flush

Figure 12. The mechanism of the hot flush

Vaginal symptoms

Vaginal itching and other changes are troubling symptoms experienced by many women. Vaginal symptoms may not appear until several years after menopause, and they are a direct result of a lack of oestrogen. The vulvar skin, fat and tissues are particuarly sensitive to oestrogen: when hormone levels drop, after a few years the skin and tissue may begin to atrophy or shrink. But vaginal dryness is an early sympton of the menopause in many women. The external genitalia become smaller and pubic hair thins. The vagina also shrinks, and the tissue lining it thins out. Vaginal secretions become less acid and make the woman more prone to vaginitis, resulting in burning and itching. Many women also find that sexual intercourse becomes painful – a particularly distressing symptom since so many women worry that they will lose their sexual appeal as they grow older.

Studies have found that the vaginal symptoms are not as pronounced in women who have frequent intercourse and/or orgasms (defined as intercourse three or more times a month and orgasm at least once a week). Of course, this may be difficult for some women who lack sexual partners, or who already are troubled by vaginal symptoms. Sometime the itching, burning and painful intercourse can be relieved by using a lubricating cream or ointment. But often oestrogen is needed, taken either orally or in the form of a cream, suppository or skin patch.

Urinary tract

Lack of oestrogen may cause changes in the urethra and bladder, making a woman more vulnerable to cystitis. A tipping of the bladder – usually the result of muscle weakness or damage from earlier childbirth – may exacerbate stress incontinence or other bladder control problems.

Palpitations

Many women complain of a rapid heartbeat, or palpitations, during menopause. The palpitations are sometimes accompanied by hot flushes, but at other times occur independently. The rapid heartbeat is believed to be caused by the same vasomotor irregularity that triggers the hot flushes. The palpitations are harmless, but can be frightening and troubling. If palpitations are troublesome, they usually can be stopped by taking a low dose of a beta blocker, a drug

110

that is often prescribed to treat angina and high blood pressure but it has other side effects you should ask about.

Mood swings

Periods of irritability, crying spells, depression and other mood changes are common. They may be a combination of organic causes or rooted in emotional upheavals. Middle age is a time of change and reassessment for both men and women. By this time, children are growing up and leaving home. Career opportunities may be dwindling or at least levelling off. People also begin to notice undeniable signs of getting older: parents age and die, the mirror reveals new wrinkles and greying hair, and they no longer have the stamina of youth. Coming to terms with these changes can be depressing, especially in today's youth-oriented society.

Swelling

Many women complain of abdominal swelling, often accompanied by intestinal wind. The swelling is caused by fluid retention, and is similar to pre-menstrual swelling or that which occurs in early pregnancy.

The cause of pre-menstrual and pregnancy swelling is not known, but it is probably due to hormonal changes. Reducing salt intake, avoiding tight-fitting clothing and foods that provoke wind may lessen the discomfort. If swelling persists or is troublesome, a mild diuretic may be prescribed.

Weight gain

At about the time of menopause, most women notice that they are adding a little extra weight, often around the abdomen, leading to middle-age spread.

As we grow older, our metabolism slows down and we do not burn up as many calories as before. Most people do not adjust their food intake according to their lowered energy needs, so, unless they increase their physical activity, they will gain weight.

This is concentrated in the abdominal area because fat here is more mobile. People with excessive abdominal fat have higher levels of blood cholesterol, blood glucose and a greater risk of heart attack.

Poor muscle tone also may add to abdominal sagging, particularly in women who have had children. Toning exercises can bring them back into shape, but many women neglect these exercises after pregnancy. As they lose weight, they become less conscious of their sagging muscles, only to rediscover them years later when they add a few extra kilogrammes/pounds.

Finally, oestrogen causes weight gain in some women. Birth control pills with a relatively high oestrogen content cause weight gain in some women and oestrogen replacement therapy during menopause can have the same effect. But even women who do not take oestrogen may gain abdominal weight. This is believed to be due to androgens, which promote abdominal fat deposits in both men and women.

Sexuality

Some women find that menopause decreases their interest in and enjoyment of sex, while others find that their sexual desire and responsiveness increases. These change may be due to a combination of psychological and hormonal factors. At about this time of life, many women experience the loss of a sexual partner, either through death or divorce. A partner may be going through his own midlife crisis or have other problems that reduce his sexual interest or capabilities. As is so often emphasized, sexuality is a fragile thing that requires considerable attention and practice to keep alive, enjoyable and exciting. Thus, it is virtually impossible to separate the physical and emotional aspects of sex.

The dryness and thinning of vaginal tissue result in painful intercourse, negating any pleasure, and many couples find they avoid sex simply because it is uncomfortable for the woman.

Contraception and worries about possible pregnancy may also be a factor; although fertility is lessened as ovulation becomes more infrequent, as long as a woman is ovulating, pregnancy is possible.

Selecting an appropriate form of birth control can be troubling for an older woman and sterilisation is now more common. But thousands rely on reversible methods, with the pill being the most popular. Many doctors feel, however, that women over the age of 40 should not use the combination pill because of the increased risk of high blood pressure, clotting and heart disease that comes with age. In addition, women over the age of 35 who smoke should not take the pill, since this may increase the risk of vascular disease. The mini- or progestogen-only pill is more appropriate for older women, but it causes a higher incidence of irregular or breakthrough bleeding. IUDs need to be considered in the light of the recent debate about them.

Since ovulation is erratic among most menopausal women, rhythm or other so-called natural methods of birth control are even more unreliable. This leaves barrier methods, such as the condom, diaphragm or vaginal sponge, as about the only alternative means of birth control.

Of course, after menopause is firmly established (a year or more since the last menstrual period), birth control is no longer a worry, and many post-menopausal women find this a liberating factor that actually enhances their sex lives. Also, after menopause, women have high levels of androgens – male hormones that are secreted by the adrenal glands and, in part, converted to oestrogen in fatty tissue. The androgens also serve to increase libido, which explains why many menopausal women actually experience a heightened interest in sex.

Artificial menopause

An ever increasing number of women never go through natural menopause; instead, they have a total hysterectomy (which includes removal of the ovaries) that prematurely ends their menstruating years. In recent decades, there has been mounting controversy over the number of hysterectomies performed in many countries, with the focus springing from a Boston study. This appeared to show that women in one area had higher numbers of hysterectomies compared to those in another area, this being due to a difference in surgeons' attitudes, rather than the women's needs. More than 800,000 American women have hysterectomies each year, and up to a third or more of these have been called unnecessary. American women are up to four times more likely to have a hysterectomy than are women in other industrialised countries. In the UK the approach has generally been more cautious, but still a cause for close attention.

Some doctors honestly feel that removal of the uterus, ovaries and other reproductive organs lessens a woman's chance of developing cancer. If she no longer plans to have children, and there are signs that point to a future risk, why not simply do a hysterectomy? This argument ignores the trauma of hysterectomy; sexuality is affected, especially if the operation is a total hysterectomy (removal of the cervix and upper part of the vagina). Many hysterectomies today are total, as opposed to subtotal, which entails removal of only the uterus.

Of course, if the ovaries are also removed, the woman immediately

113

loses her female hormones and goes into an abrupt menopause that may carry more severe symptoms than a later, natural menopause. Some doctors recommend that the ovaries be removed during a hysterectomy if the woman is 40 or older, reasoning that she will probably go into menopause in a few years anyway and that this spares her the risk of ovarian cancer. This argument can be countered by the fact that the risk of ovarian cancer is low – about 1 per cent for women of 40. Also, the average age of menopause is still 51; a 40-year-old woman who has had her ovaries removed may have had more than a decade remaining of natural hormonal production. This is important, because women who lose their ovaries at an early age have a much higher risk of osteoporosis – a thinning of the bones. There is also evidence that the risk of a heart attack also rises.

In general, there are three indications for a hysterectomy: (1) cancer of the reproductive organs; (2) severe infection, or disease of the fallopian tubes or ovaries that cannot be treated by other means; (3) large fibroid tumors that are causing other problems and cannot be removed on their own.

If a woman has any doubt about the need for a hysterectomy, she should get a second opinion. Questionable reasons for which a hysterectomy may be recommended include small, symptomless fibroids; bleeding that can be treated by other less drastic means; pelvic pain; prolapse of the uterus; and abnormal cervical smears that are not clearly cancer. In the past in some countries, hysterectomies have been done as a sterilisation procedure, on the grounds that if the woman is going to be sterilised, she might as well have a hysterectomy so she can avoid having periods and reduce her risk of uterine cancer. This is no longer considered justification for a hysterectomy.

Of course, there are instances in which a hysterectomy is the preferred treatment. There is no question if uterine or cervical cancer has been diagnosed. A woman who is severely anaemic because she bleeds profusely for eight or nine days every month may indeed require a hysterectomy. The same may not be true of a woman who has heavy periods but is otherwise healthy; she may be treated with birth control pills or other more conservative means.

· A hysterectomy because of a fibroid tumour may or may not be justified, depending upon the circumstances. Fibroid tumours are made up of smooth muscle cells and are also called myomas or leiomyomas (myos means 'muscle', leios means 'smooth'). They are most common after the age of 30 or 35, with a prevalence of up to 50 per cent in some ethnic groups. Most are small and slow-growing. They very rarely develop into malignant cancers, and many women have fibroids without experiencing symptoms. There is no reason to do a hysterectomy because of these small, symptomless fibroids, which are actually a variant of what is normal.

A large, fast-growing fibroid that causes pain, bleeding, fertility problems and abdominal swelling is a different story, and there are circumstances in which it should be removed. If left untreated, this type of fibroid can grow very large – some fibroids weighing more than 45kg (100lb) have been recorded. Fortunately, this is very rare. More commonly, the woman will look as though she is several months pregnant.

Removal can sometimes be done surgically without taking out the uterus. The operation, called a myomectomy, entails making an incision in the uterine wall and cutting out the fibroid. It is a more complicated operation than a hysterectomy, and, not uncommonly, the fibroid will grow back. Still, a myomectomy is the preferred operation for a younger woman who wants to have a child, or for a woman who is experiencing fertility problems because of fibroids.

Hormone replacement therapy

The use of oestrogen replacement therapy following menopause has been the subject of considerable controversy in recent years. On one side are the endocrinologists and others who contend that, following menopause, women experience an abnormal oestrogen deficiency. (At one time, a womans's average life span did not extend many years beyond menopause, but today, a woman may expect to live another 30 years or more in this oestrogen-deficient state.) On the other side are people who feel that menopause is a normal stage, and thus the hormonal changes that accompany it also are normal. Mounting evidence of the reduced incidence of hip fractures and of heart disease in women who have had HRT supports the rationale for this therapy. New ways of combining oestrogen and progesterone to mimic the body's normal levels of these two hormones are increasing its safety. There have been recent studies that have have been questioning the relationship between HRT and the incidence of breast cancer.

The therapy has developed this century as the production of the various compounds of oestrogen has grown. Millions of women now take oestrogen to ease menopausal symptoms, particularly hot flushes and vaginal dryness, and to help prevent osteoporosis, which is so common among older women.

Despite the fact the many women suffer from symptoms that can be eased by oestrogen replacement, many are reluctant to take it, and their doctors hesitant to prescribe it. A large part of this is due to outdated research. In the US in the 1950s and 1960s oestrogen replacement was prescribed for many women going through menopause. The unrealistic promise of 'forever feminine' (interpreted to mean 'forever young') led many women to believe that if they took oestrogen, they not only would get rid of their hot flushes and other troubling symptoms, but their skin wrinkles and other signs of ageing as well. Obviously, oestrogen cannot stop the clock, and it is not a miraculous 'fountain of youth', but it may help maintain bones and perhaps protect against heart disease – important benefits which some US doctors in the 1960s and early 1970s felt justified the routine, long-term use of hormone replacement. Then came several disturbing reports in the mid-1970s that women on continuous long-term oestrogen replacement had a higher risk of endometrial cancer.

This changed the pattern of oestrogen replacement prescribing in number and dosage. The cancer scare quickly reached the women themselves, who, understandably, reasoned that it was better to endure hot flushes than to risk cancer. As with other areas in medicine, more caution, research and knowledge among doctors has perhaps caused the pendulum to stay more in the middle. The fact is you can abolish the cancer risk by adding a progestogen, although this means the woman will have regular, withrawal bleeding. Doctors need to know and inform women of the balance of risk. A lack of oestrogen replacement can cause problems that are more serious than the relatively slight risk of endometrial cancer.

In recent years, we have become increasingly aware of the seriousness of osteoporosis. Many older women can expect to suffer at least one broken bone, largely as a consequence of osteoporosis and fractures or other complications of osteoporosis contribute to thousands of deaths. This is many times the number of women at risk of dying from endometrial cancer. A woman breaks a hip or leg bone, is hospitalised for surgery, and then during the prolonged bed rest, may develop a blood clot that lodges in the lung, infection, pneumonia or some other complication that results in death.

Bone thinning is a gradual process that is thought to begin when a woman is in her thirties and accelerates sharply following menopause.

The risk of osteoporosis is particularly pronounced in women whose ovaries have never functioned or whose ovaries were removed at an early age. Therefore, oestrogen replacement is especially important for a woman who has a hysterectomy, in which the ovaries are removed, before the age of 40. Other factors that increase the risk of osteoporosis include cigarette smoking, which affects oestrogen metabolism, and a diet deficient in calcium and vitamin D. People who are fine-boned – for example, white women of northern European extraction and Orientals – have more osteoporosis than those with more bone mass, such as black women. Hormonal imbalances or diseases that upset calcium metabolism also can cause osteoporosis. If you are on replacement therapy, then smoking and alcohol will also reduce its effectiveness.

For reasons that are not completely understood, oestrogen seems to help maintain bone strength and prevent further thinning from osteoporosis. Hormone therapy does not reverse the process, although there often is an improvement in the early years of oestrogen therapy.

Oestrogen has a protective effect on a woman's cardiovascular system. Coronary disease and heart attacks are relatively uncommon among pre-menopausal women. The hormones act directly on the blood vessels in a way beneficial to your whole circulation. In the decade or two following menopause, women gradually begin to catch up with men in developing heart disease, and, among older women, it is a leading cause of death. A number of factors in addition to oestrogen may account for the sexual differences in heart disease. Until relatively recently, cigarette smoking – one of the major risk factors for a heart attack – has not been as common in women as in men. Nor have women been as subjected to stress in the workplace. This is changing, but it is too early to tell whether women are experiencing a concomitant rise in early heart attacks.

The mechanism whereby oestrogen may protect the heart is unknown, although some experts feel that it involves cholesterol metabolism. Following menopause, the average woman's cholesterol level goes up. The level of LDL cholesterol – the type that contributes to the buildup of fatty deposits in the arteries – also rises. Oestrogen replacement prevents the rise in total and LDL cholesterol that often occurs after menopause, which may explain its protective effect.

Recent studies at Erasmus University in Rotterdam indicate that oestrogen replacement may also help prevent rheumatoid arthritis among older women. They found a two-thirds reduction in rheumatoid arthritis among women taking oestrogen. The hormone may be supressing the inflammation that damages the joints. Or the post-menopausal hormone therapy may somehow mimic the protection against the disease seen among pregnant women, who routinely enjoy a remission in rheumatoid arthritis.

Endocrinologists are convinced that the benefits of hormone replacement therapy outweigh the risks. Many doctors now feel that the judicious use of hormones, during and after menopause, not only eases the immediate symptoms, but also has potential long-term benefits in maintaining bones and perhaps protecting against heart attacks. Still, women on hormone therapy should be particularly diligent about having regular check-ups, which should include a cervical smear every six months.

The issue, perhaps, is convincing doctors and women to learn more about the role of hormones and therapy and to weigh the risk factors against benefits. The lack of a consistent 'model' regime and therapy which are acceptable to women, is also an obstacle.

Over the last decade, there has been an increasing trend toward both oestrogen and progestogen replacement, thereby mimicking what happens during a normal cycle. Taken alone, oestrogen causes a buildup of the uterine lining, or endometrium. Some authorities believe this unchallenged proliferation of endometrial tissue is what increases the risk of cancer. By taking an oestrogen for 20 days and adding a progestogen for 10 of them, a woman will have a shedding of the excess endometrial tissue when she stops both pills for five days – similar to what happens in a menstrual period. Some endocrinologists also note that addition of progestogen also may help prevent excessive hormonal stimulation of the breasts. Although there is no strong evidence that oestrogen replacement causes breast cancer, there are some types of cancer that are stimulated by hormones. Women who have had breast cancer with positive oestrogen receptors are not advised to take oestrogen replacement therapy.

Some women may experience adverse side effects from hormone therapy, although this is relatively rare in the low doses used for long-term replacement therapy. Symptoms may include nausea, vomiting, swelling, weight gain, breast tenderness, headaches, dizziness, increased susceptibility to vaginal yeast infections and breakthrough vaginal bleeding. These adverse reactions usually subside and disappear in two or three months, but if they persist or are severe, a lower dosage may be tried.

Conjugated oestrogens are the most commonly used to treat menopausal symptoms. They can be taken orally or applied directly to the vagina in a topical cream. In a typical course of treatment a woman will take it daily for 20 days (a higher dosage may be given if hot flushes persist or if there is progressive osteoporosis), and then a progestogen for 10 days, then nothing for the next five days. The progestogen should be followed by light bleeding. (This ends in about two years for half of women treated.) She then starts a new course. Another way is to take the oestrogen and progestogen in a low dose every day. This does not cause the uterus lining to be shed and the low dose progestogen may help protect the uterus against cancer.

There also is a newer method of administering oestrogen through slow release from a patch on the skin. The patch is changed twice a week, and progestogen pills are taken orally. The main advantage of the patch is that it delivers a low, steady dosage of the hormone, and one therefore not as likely to produce adverse side effects as the pills, which give a larger dosage all at once. It also bypasses the liver metabolism and avoids fat changes in the blood which influence blood pressure. Early studies seem to indicate that the patch has the same protective benefits as oral forms.

Any unscheduled vaginal bleeding is a warning sign to see a doctor as soon as possible. This applies to all women, especially after menopause. Vaginal bleeding is the major sign of cervical and uterine cancers and the incidence of these cancers increases markedly with menopause. Before menopause is established, many women tend to have irregular bleeding. It may be difficult to tell if this bleeding is a period or a warning sign to see a doctor. So err on the side of caution. All women should have pelvic examination and cervical smear at least annually with approach of menopause (as well as an annual breast examination and mammogram), and more often if they are on hormone therapy.

Some doctors recommend weaning a woman off hormone replacement after two to five years, unless she has osteoporosis. Others feel that, so long as there are no contraindications, the hormones can be continued for life. The important thing is to have your course tailored to you. The major side effects of oestrogens are salt and water retention, which can cause swelling, nausea and breast soreness.

Synthetic, as opposed to natural oestrogens can promote a

tendency for blood to clot, but the dosages given in replacement therapy should be so low that this is not likely. Women who have a history of abnormal clotting, which can lead to development of thrombophlebitis (the formation of a clot in a vein), or a thromboembolism (a piece of clot that breaks away and travels through the circulation to the lungs, heart, brain or other vital organ) are not candidates for hormone replacement therapy. Thrombophlebitis freqently occurs as a complication of pelvic surgery; a woman undergoing an operation in this area should stop taking the hormones well in advance of the surgery to minimise the risk of abnormal clotting. Diabetes should be checked for before hormone replacement. In addition, a woman with a history of a previous stroke or heart attack should not take these hormones.

Beyond hormone therapy

Although hormone replacement is important to a woman's health and wellbeing during and after menopause, it is not a panacea. How well we cope with and adjust to mid-life changes depends more upon our emotional health and feelings of self-esteem than our hormones. Hormones can relieve the physical symptoms that come with the menopause, and probably have a protective effect against some of the ravages of old age. But they will not solve problems of the mind and soul.

PART III

Endocrine Disorders

CHAPTER SEVEN

Osteoporosis and Other Diseases Related to Calcium Metabolism

Despite the new awareness the public has about the problems of bones getting thinner (osteoporosis) particularly in old age, there are still many misconceptions about the condition and the roles of calcium in maintaining health.

Importance of calcium

Calcium provides the foundation for strong bones and teeth. It is also important in the functioning of muscles, nerves, endocrine and exocrine glands, hormones and other body tissue. Calcium helps to bind cells together, activate enzymes and promote blood clotting and fertilisation. It may also be useful in the treatment of high blood pressure and may help protect against cancer of the colon.

Calcium is by far the most abundant mineral in the body. The average adult woman has about 875g (1lb 14oz) and an adult man about 1kg (2.2lb). Of this 99 per cent is in the bones and teeth; the remainder circulates in the blood with about ten grams being in the body tissues.

Calcium metabolism is a complex process that involves several organ systems and hormones. Food provides calcium, with the best sources being milk, milk products, fish and green leafy vegetables (see Table 5). A certain amount of calcium is lost in the urine and faeces every day.

Although most people think of bones as being composed of inert, static tissue, they are actually in a constant state of remodelling. Since the bones serve as the body's storehouse for calcium, they release the mineral in response to hormonal signals when calcium blood levels fall, and then reabsorb it to maintain strength and density. When the level of blood calcium falls to a certain point, the parathyroid glands secrete parathyroid hormone into the bloodstream. This signals the kidneys to return calcium, which would ordinarily be excreted in urine, to the blood instead and causes the bones to release some of their calcium. It also stimulates the conversion of vitamin D to its active form, the hormone 25 hydroxycholecalciferol. This hormone promotes absorption of dietary calcium from the intestine, and also increases the kidneys' reabsorption of the mineral.

Table 5: Calcium Content of Foods (Mg per 100g)

Skim milk, dried	1190
Whole milk	120
Cheddar cheese	800
Cottage cheese	60
Parmesan	1220
Sardines	550
Pilchards, canned	300
Whitebait	860
Cod, fried	80
Figs, dried	280
Currants	95
Almonds	250
Brazils	180
Broccoli, boiled	65
Spinach, boiled	330
Red cabbage, raw	76

A third hormone, calcitonin, secreted by the thyroid, acts as a calcium-sparing substance to prevent excessive breakdown of bone tissue. Oestrogen also protects the bones from excessive calcium loss by stimulating the secretion of calcitonin and promoting the conversion of vitamin D, as well as by other mechanisms not fully understood. In contrast, cortisone causes bone loss, a factor which limits its use in arthritis, other inflammatory disorders and asthma. Growth hormone increases bone formation, and thyroid deficiency in children causes stunted growth while an excess in children or adults causes bone loss. Other factors affecting bone remodelling include:

Exercise
Like muscles, bones respond to the stress of exercise by growing larger and stronger. It increases the flow of blood to bones and so may affect hormonal balance.

Tobacco, alcohol and medicines
We do not know why but women smokers tend to have more osteoporosis. Tobacco may lower oestrogen levels. Heavy coffee drinkers are also more likely to become osteoporotic. If you are fond of coffee, cut down to a few cups a day or drink decaffeinated. Excessive intake of alcohol interferes with the intestines' ability to absorb calcium. Young alcoholics often have serious bone loss, but the cause may be different from that of tobacco. Steroids, diuretics, aluminium-containing antacids, thyroid supplements and anti-convulsant drugs can interfere with calcium metabolism and cause bone loss.

Fluoridation
Fluoride added to water can help maintain strong teeth and appears to have a similar effect on bones. It may be used as part of a treatment for osteoporosis and other bone disorders. There is a long and well-documented debate about the levels of fluoride additives in water.

Dietary factors
The old Greek adage of 'nothing to excess' holds good here. Different countries go through extreme swings for and against certain foods and diets and you need to keep a middle course despite advertisers, and that includes drug companies working away at the medical profession. The World Health Organization recommends up to 400–500mg per day of calcium for an adult man or woman; a pregnant or lactating woman needs over 1000mg a day of calcium. You also need phosphorus which hardens the bones. But a high-meat diet, and similar high phosphorus, protein-rich foods (soft drinks may be rich in phosphorus), can cause bone loss if there is excess intake. Excessive salt can increase your blood pressure and cause calcium excretion by the kidneys, as can four or more cups of coffee containing

caffeine. Too much roughage can hinder calcium absorption from the intestines. Oxalates in spinach, rhubarb, asparagus, beets, and some other green vegetables bind to calcium and prevent its absorption.

The very common habit of taking of extra vitamins in the US is also spreading to other countries, so it needs to be said that excessive intake of vitamins A or D stimulates bone loss, though a deficiency of vitamin D results in rickets in which the bones soften.

Osteoporosis

This mean porous bones and is caused by a loss of calcium, making them thin and brittle. It is primarily a condition in women and perhaps one out of four women over the age of 60 suffers from it. So do half of all women who have had surgically induced menopause. Most do not know they have it until they break a bone, most frequently a hip or vertebra, and by then it is usually quite advanced, with considerable bone loss, although all bones become thinner with age. Perhaps a third of women in their sixties suffer fractures.

There are two basic kinds of bone tissue, the outer cortical bone which is dense and hard, and the inner trabecular bone, which looks like a honeycomb. Your spine's vertebrae are mostly trabecular bone enclosed in a thin shell of cortical, while the legs are mainly cortical with trabecular bone at the ends. The honeycomb has more surface area to release calcium and so is also most vulnerable to osteoporosis. You begin to lose small amounts of the trabecular bone from your mid-twenties, while cortical continues to build until the mid-thirties when it begins to decline gradually.

Women lose bone faster than men after menopause because of the reduced oestrogen, perhaps at twice the speed, and particularly in the first five or six years. It is not unusual for women with osteoporosis to lose eight or more inches from their adult height through the bone loss and as the vertebrae collapse. It is a slow and almost unnoticeable process but a woman will notice that her waist is thicker (though weight is perhaps the same) and clothes no longer fit. If several vertebrae collapse in rapid succession it is, of course, more noticeable with 5–7.5cm (2–3in) loss in height within a few months.

At the time of collapse there may be severe back pain, perhaps becoming chronic because of muscle spasms caused by inflammation around the collapsing vertebrae. A curve may develop in the spine, the classic 'widow's hump'. A woman may break a wrist bone or hip

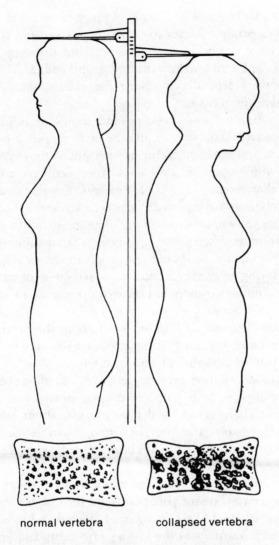

normal vertebra   collapsed vertebra

Figure 13. Height loss of 7.5–20cm (3–8in) is not unusual in advanced osteoporosis

in a minor fall, although there are instances where there is no apparent reason for the fracture. In fact she may remember a sharp pain which caused her to fall, the fracture preceding the 'accident'.

Hip fractures may leave a woman disabled for the rest of her life. About 15 per cent die shortly after the accident and 30 per cent within a year due to complications such as a blood clot that causes a stroke

127

or heart attack. This is why there is so much room for improved preventive work around homes to make them safer and suited to the elderly through easier working and walking surfaces, safer bathrooms and cupboards, hand rails and grab handles. They not only help maintain independence among the elderly but save a lot of trauma and hospital costs.

When looking at bone building and decline it is important to realise that at a certain stage in life the body reaches a peak in bone mass. This is an important factor in determining the degree of osteoporosis in women (and in some men, since men have a higher peak bone mass than women). It is the fall off after this that matters.

Early growth and the periods of pregnancy and breastfeeding all require large amounts of calcium. The more your body needs calcium, the more it can take – if it gets it. So, making sure you get enough at the right time should not be left to chance. High levels of oestrogen during pregnancy stimulate the activation of vitamin D and increase calcium absorption and the extra progestogen has a protective effect on the bones.

The experts are still finding out a lot about this whole area and views differ. Some suggest that bone loss may be due to widespread calcium deficiency and that menopausal women should have a daily intake of 1500mg. Earlier remarks in this book, about oestrogen replacement following menopause to counter osteoporosis, should be remembered. There was also debate in 1989 about the risk that, should therapy stop later on, the osteoporosis would accelerate. Some experts say this evidence has been refuted, but there do seem to be differences in expert opinion.

We also need to think about bone maintenance throughout life and while it may be too late for you, that is not the case for your children or those in your care! Exercise, reduced alcohol and tobacco intake, and hereditary warnings in the history of parents and grandparents can all help you plan. A thin, small-boned woman is more at risk than a heavy-set, large-boned one. Other possible signs of susceptibility include thin, transparent skin, especially on the hands and loosening of the teeth.

Diagnosis
Since the development of osteoporosis is gradual, and not easy to spot at a single point in time, early diagnosis is essential. X-rays only show a problem when about 30 per cent of bone has been lost. Mineral

analysis can detect it accurately but equipment is only available at special centres. In fact your much under-rated dentist may be your best ally, because jaw X-rays taken over a few years may show a decline in bone mass; loosening of the teeth may indicate the same.

Treatment
Prevention of further loss and restoration of bone are the main aims of treatment. It is better to start tackling this problem, if it is developing, early in a woman's fifties when you can put something back. Left until your stature has significantly shortened and a hump is develop ing means there is only the possibility of stopping further deterioration and not reversing some of the bone loss. A typical course of treatment involves hormone replacement therapy, exercise, calcium supplements, plus perhaps vitamin D or alpha-calcidol, an activated form of vitamin D. Sometimes fluoride may be included in severe cases and it is the only medication that appears to increase bone mass, though in relatively few patients. A third may have severe side effects. Such new bone may be more brittle and vulnerable to fractures, and, while the spine may benefit, you may lose bone at the hips.

Calcitonin hormone from the thyroid has been used experimentally and has shown an easing of symptoms as well as small increases in bone tissue, though the effects are temporary. However it has to be given by injection and there have been unfortunate side effects. There is a nasal preparation being tried out and this may be more acceptable after full evaluation.

It is very important to analyse your diet and lifestyle because significant changes in the way you live can create marked benefits for your body.

Other disorders of calcium metabolism

Blood levels of calcium that are too low (hypocalcaemia) can cause tetany, muscle convulsions, commonly in the forearm, hands and wrist, seizures, mental and emotional disturbances, malabsorption problems, abdominal pain, constipation and diarrhoea. If it continues for a long time it can produce abnormalities in the skin, hair, nails, teeth and the lens of the eye (cataracts). You may lose eyebrow, eyelash, pubic and underarm hair, while nails become thin, brittle and develop grooves. Teeth may develop yellow spots and grooves. Conditions such as eczema and psoriasis may worsen.

A lack of vitamin D may often be the commonest cause of hypocalcaemia and this has been pinpointed amongst vegans and certain ethnic groups because of their dietary habits. Other causes of hypocalcaemia include kidney disease, cirrhosis of the liver, low parathyroid hormone or accidental damage to the parathyroid glands after neck surgery, certain cancers, tumours that secrete calcitonin, pancreatitis and magnesium deficiency. Sometimes premature babies are born with hypocalcaemia but it usually disappears within a period of a week or two.

Acute tetany can be eased by injections of calcium and then pill supplements, often with activated vitamin D. But the underlying cause should be identified.

Too much calcium, hypercalcaemia, is almost always a sign of a serious underlying condition, though excess alkali intake is perhaps commoner than generally appreciated.

In general, many of the symptoms of hypercalcaemia are vague and could be caused by a number of other illnesses. Such symptoms include fatigue, lethargy, muscle weakness, loss of appetite, nausea and vomiting, weight loss, constipation, headaches and mental changes. More specific symptoms which would indicate hypercalcaemia include thirst, excessive urination and dehydration. If it is allowed to progress it causes uncontrolled vomiting, severe dehydration, mental disturbances or unconsciousness and, finally, death from widespread tissue destruction and calcification. This is rare.

About 80 per cent of hypercalcaemia cases are caused either by excessive production of parathyroid hormone or as a result of complications of cancer – especially multiple myeloma, lymphoma, leukaemia, or advanced cancers of the breast, lung and kidney. Other causes include vitamin D deficiency, thyroid disease, sarcoidosis (a rare disease resembling tuberculosis) and adrenal insufficiency. Hypercalcaemia may result from being immobilised, eg in a plaster cast, if the person was in a high bone-turnover state, as would be a child. Thiazide diuretics used to treat high blood pressure may cause high calcium levels.

Treatment of hypercalcaemia means tackling the underlying disorder, giving adequate fluids to overcome dehydration and correcting the chemical imbalances it causes in the body. So, potassium depletion is common with elevated calcium and needs to be corrected. Steroids may be given to lower calcium and other drugs which work faster may be used in an emergency situation.

130

Osteomalacia and rickets

Osteomalacia is the softening of the bones due to a lack of the mineralisation which would normally give bone tissue its hardness. If the osteomalacia occurs during periods of growth, the cartilage will also be affected, causing rickets with its characteristic bowed legs, thickening at the ends of long bones, pigeon breast and other deformities.

Traditionally, osteomalacia and rickets are caused by vitamin D deficiency which stops the body using calcium, and it is usually prevented by vitamin D being added to milk and baby formula and other foods. It will also occur in kidney disorders, or where there has been removal of the stomach, where there is intestinal malabsorption, in the use of anti-convulsant drugs in children or excessive aluminium gels in adults, or when there is a genetic defect in which the body does not utilise vitamin D and phosphate. There has been an increase in both conditions in ethnic communities, particularly from the Indian subcontinent, partly due to lack of sunlight, which is needed to promote vitamin D, and partly due to diet.

Adolescent ballerinas, with delayed periods due to undernutrition, may lack the oestrogen necessary to lay down bone during the adolescent growth spurt, because they are under pressure to stay slim. These girls have a higher prevalence of scoliosis and fractures.

Bone softening and deformities can usually be prevented by early diagnosis and correction of the underlying cause. Rickets in young babies is not always apparent however, only showing up in the deformities and a failure to grow. Treatment is usually by giving large amounts of vitamin D, often with phosphorus supplements, to promote hardening of the bones. It is more complicated if kidney disease is causing the problem and in such instances removal of the parathyroid glands may be indicated.

Kidney stones

The body's inability to metabolise calcium quite often results in the development of kidney stones. Passing a kidney stone causes the most excruciating pain. They are more common among women and in 90 per cent of cases the cause is unknown. In 10 per cent it may be structural problems in the kidneys, gout, excessive parathyroid hormone or intestinal disorders. They may be made up of calcium or uric acid due to too much of these in the urine even though blood levels will be normal. If you pass a kidney stone, keep it for analysis.

There is a debate about the traditional strategy of eliminating calcium-rich foods from the diet of sufferers. The problem is not so much an excessive intake of calcium as the body's inability to properly metabolise it. Protein intake reduction, so reducing excretion in the urine of calcium, uric acid and phosphorus may be a better approach. Increasing fluid intake to dilute the urine as much as possible is also important. But take care that you do not use bottled mineral water with a high mineral content or if you live in an area where the tap water is heavily mineralised. You could be increasing your intake without realising.

In the case of calcium stones a diuretic drug may be prescribed and allopurinol, often taken by gout patients, will help prevent the formation of uric acid stones.

While stones may remain in the kidneys unnoticed, the problem occurs when one gets lodged in the ureters which take fluid from the kidneys into the bladder. This causes pain and can cause fluid back pressure in the kidneys after a few days. A cystoscope and catheter with a basketlike tip may be used to try to snare it out, and a newer treatment is to beam shock waves at the stone to disintegrate it. This is better than surgery for all concerned.

Summing up

The large number of women affected by osteoporosis means that there is growing research internationally, which should bring improved treatments. For example, OD14, which is licenced in the Netherlands, has a marked protective effect on bone mineral content and alleviates hot flushes. In Belgium researchers suggest that another drug, tiludronate, is very specific in halting bone loss without serious side effects on other systems in the body. There are many such developments, which should lead to more targeted approaches with a lower risk of side effects.

CHAPTER EIGHT

Hormones and the Breast

We are born seeking out our mother's breast, but the attraction does not end with weaning; from the cradle to the grave, both men and women are preoccupied with the female breast. A woman's breasts are universally viewed as a symbol of beauty, sexuality and nurturing – the very essence of femininity. Anything that threatens a breast takes on a significance of its own. A mastectomy because of cancer, for example, is almost as dreaded as the disease itself. This dread of losing a breast has prevented many women who suspect they have breast cancer from seeking early medical treatment – a delay that can have tragic consequences. Fortunately, this is changing as women become more involved in treatment decisions and more knowledgeable about their bodies and health.

Normal breast anatomy and function

The breast is a glandular organ designed to produce milk. In women, each breast contains about 20 lobes arranged around the nipple (see Figure 14). Each lobe branches into a number of lobules, which give rise to tiny milk-producing bulbs called acini. A network of ducts connects the lobe and its milk-producing structures to the nipple.

The nipple is surrounded by a pigmented area, the areola, which contains the sebaceous Montgomery glands. These secrete the oily substance that lubricates the nipple and sometimes they resemble small pimples. Some women mistakenly think they are abnormal growths, but they are really a normal part of the breast. Nipples also

133

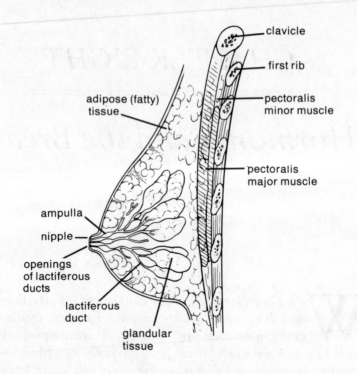

Figure 14. The normal breast

contain erectile tissue, which causes them to stand out when they are stimulated or exposed to the cold.

Breasts are very sensitive to hormones. This is often evident at birth. Many babies are born with enlarged breasts due to high levels of oestrogen, prolactin and other hormones that circulate in the mother's blood during pregnancy. As these hormones are dissipated from the baby's body, its breast tissue shrinks and remains quiescent until puberty, when the rise in sex hormones stimulates the breasts to 'bud' and start growing. Normally, only women develop breasts, but there are circumstances in which men's breasts enlarge. Pubescent boys sometimes develop enlarged breasts. They usually subside in a year or two, but can be very embarrassing to a young boy. Men who are markedly overweight may appear to develop breasts but it is fat. Certain drugs can also stimulate breast development.

Almost all adolescent girls are concerned about their breasts – that they are developing unevenly, are too big, too small, the nipples look strange, and on and on. Despite magazine ads to the contrary, there is not much, short of surgery, that we can do about the size and shape of our breasts. Breast size and contour are determined by heredity, weight and the amount of glandular tissue present. Very small breasts can be enlarged and very large ones can be reduced by plastic surgery. But this should be a last resort and is not recommended until adulthood. Frequently, having a baby or simply gaining or losing weight can have a major effect on breast size.

There are no creams, exercises or other remedies that can increase breast size. Body-building exercises can increase the size of underlying muscles and make the breasts look larger, but since the breasts themselves have no muscles, exercise will not make them bigger. Hormones can stimulate the breasts to grow, as evidenced by the fact that women taking birth control pills sometimes experience breast enlargement. But hormones should not be taken specifically to increase breast size because of the high risk of adverse side effects.

Breasts normally change with age. The developing breast is firm and the tissue is dense. During pregnancy, the breasts grow considerably, often doubling in size. As women grow older, their breasts feel lumpier. Following menopause, the lumpiness subsides and the breasts become softer and less glandular. There is a reduction in fatty tissue, and the supporting ligaments and skin lose some of their elasticity. These changes are not as pronounced in women who take hormone replacement.

Except during pregnancy, breasts are usually their fullest during young adulthood, but this varies considerably. Some women are relatively flat-chested until they have had a baby, and are pleasantly surprised to find that they retain some of the size added during pregnancy. Others end up with smaller breasts after pregnancy. Some women mistakenly think that nursing 'ruined' their breasts. In reality, breastfeeding has very little effect on the size or shape of breasts. This is determined by the amount of glandular tissue, and some women retain more of this tissue following pregnancy, while others have less after childbirth and nursing. Breastfeeding is highly beneficial to both the mother and child, and not an experience that should be missed because of its possible effects on breast appearance. The classic, sagging breasts of African rural women are more due to lack of bra support than breastfeeding.

How the menstrual cycle affects the breasts

During each menstrual cycle, breasts go through a series of changes that correspond with the rise and fall of hormones. The effects are most noticeable during the pre-menstrual phase, when the breasts become noticeably swollen and even tender. This swelling is due to the rise in oestrogen and progesterone during the luteal, or pre-menstrual, phase. These hormones cause increased blood flow to the breast and promote retention of body fluid; they also stimulate swelling and proliferation of the milk glands. Many women find they need a larger bra size during the pre-menstrual phase, and even the slightest touch can be painful.

Women who have fibrocystic breasts may be particularly bothered by swelling and discomfort in the pre-menstrual phase. The increased retention of fluid results in added swelling of the cysts – benign, fluid-filled sacs. Until recently, it was thought that women with fibrocystic breasts had an increased risk of breast cancer but this does not seem to be the case. Cysts do make breast self-examination difficult, however, and thus the presence of an abnormal lump might be hidden by 'normal' cysts.

With menstruation and the fall in hormones, the breast swelling subsides. About seven to 10 days after the start of menstruation, the breasts are at their smallest. This is the best time of the menstrual cycle for a woman to carefully examine her breasts, checking for any lumps, thickening, dimpling of the skin or other changes that may signal breast cancer. Even at this time in the menstrual cycle, most women will notice that their breasts have a somewhat lumpy feel. This is due to normal glandular tissue. Each woman, especially if she tends to have fibrocystic breasts, should get to know the normal feel of her breasts, so that she can be alert to a new lump or one that somehow feels different. Familiarity with the 'normal' lumps will make it easier to find abnormal ones.

Pregnancy and lactation

Breast changes are among the first signs of conception. A woman often knows that she is pregnant simply by observing what is happening to her breasts at the time when she would normally expect to have her menstrual period. The breasts become more swollen and tender than usual and the areola become darker and enlarged. The breasts feel fuller than usual, and, as the pregnancy continues, the fullness becomes more pronounced, though the tenderness character-istic of the first few weeks subsides, Even so, most women find they are more comfortable wearing a bra, and a larger size is usually needed – that provides firm support. Some women prefer to wear a bra continuously, even while sleeping.

During the last half of pregnancy there may be increased nipple discharge. This is usually in the form of clear or milky fluid, although sometimes there may be a drop or two of blood. This discharge is normal and indicates increased glandular activity resulting from the hormonal changes that are preparing the breasts to produce milk.

Breast growth during pregnancy often leaves reddish stretch marks. Apart from softening the skin, creams do little or no good. The marks never totally disappear, but usually fade with time and often are barely noticeable.

As term approaches, breast engorgement is more pronounced and there may be an increase in the nipple discharge. The breasts begin to secrete a thick, yellowish material called colostrum. This is a forerunner to milk, and is secreted for a day or two after childbirth. It is thought to contain antibodies that are important to give the newborn baby immunity, but babies who are not breastfed seem to be fine without colostrum.

The manufacture and release of breast milk is controlled by a finely tuned hormone feedback system. Shortly after the baby is born, he or she should be allowed to suckle. This breast stimulation signals the pituitary to release oxytocin. This hormone has several functions: it causes the uterus to contract, and is instrumental in labour and in the contractions that are needed to stop bleeding and restore uterine muscle tone following delivery. It also causes the milk ducts to contract and release milk to the nipple. While this is going on, the pituitary releases prolactin, the hormone that is needed to produce milk.

Most women produce enough milk for their babies. By the end of the first week after birth a nursing mother is producing about 500ml (17oz) of milk. This amount doubles by the end of the third month, and increases as the baby's needs grow. In some societies, it is common for a mother to breastfeed for two or three years, and among certain isolated tribes, women breastfeed their children until adolescence.

New mothers worry that their babies are not getting enough milk for proper growth. If the baby is gaining normally, it is safe to assume he or she is receiving enough nourishment. On average, a baby requires about 50 calories per day for each 450g (1lb) of weight. Thus a 4.5-kg (10-lb) baby will need 500 calories per day. Twenty-eight ml

(1fl oz) of breastmilk contains about 20 calories, so the baby should consume 710ml (25fl oz) of milk a day.

Many women fear that they will not be able to nurse for a variety of reasons. For example, some women have inverted nipples and worry that they will not be able to breastfeed because of them. The baby's suckling usually draws the nipples out and the woman can nurse without problems. If not, she can wear a special device that will enable the baby to nurse. Occasionally, a woman will experience sore, cracked nipples. Washing them with warm water and a mild soap before and after feeding and applying a skin oil after nursing usually solves this problem. If inflammation occurs, a physician should be contacted to ensure that infection has not set in.

Any sort of breast stimulation can cause a flow of milk. Often, simply hearing a baby's cry is enough to prompt a release of milk. Inserting a clean cloth inside the bra will absorb this milk and prevent staining of clothes.

While nursing, a woman should be careful to consume adequate calories and nutrients, especially calcium, to fulfil the needs of both her and her baby. This is probably not the best time to try to lose extra pounds that may have been added during pregnancy. The appetite and hunger centres of nursing women send out particularly strong messages, designed to ensure that a woman eats enough to make the milk needed by her baby. Breastfeeding itself uses calories and on average, a woman who breastfeeds for six months will lose 10 to 12 pounds. Since this should be a time of relaxation and enjoyment for the mother, it may be best to postpone any attempts to diet until after the baby is weaned. Otherwise, cutting back on calories requires almost superhuman willpower.

Women who breastfeed should be particularly careful about taking medicines, including the pill, antibiotics and aspirin, illicit drugs, alcohol and other substances that are potentially harmful to the baby. Nicotine and tobacco substances also enter breastmilk, as do marijuana, cocaine and other drugs. Small amounts of coffee and tea are probably not harmful but caffeine does appear in breastmilk and you may prefer to use decaffeinated brands.

Not all women can, or want, to breastfeed. If a woman decides not to breastfeed there are good powdered baby milks that provide almost complete nutrition for the baby although they cannot provide the natural immunity. A woman who knows from the beginning that she does not want to breastfeed usually will be given medication to halt milk production. Wearing a tight bra or binding the breasts to prevent nipple stimulation also helps stop milk production. When it is time to wean the baby, most women find that if they simply reduce the number of nursings per day, and finally stop, they have no trouble with continued milk production. During this weaning period a woman should refrain from breast stimulation during sex as this can promote the flow of milk.

Benign breast conditions

The majority of breast lumps turn out to be harmless. Although about 70 per cent are benign, they all need to be checked by a doctor to make sure they are not caused by cancer or some other condition requiring treatment.

Fibrocystic lumpiness is the most common benign breast condition and by 30 most women have some in their breasts. It progresses until a woman reaches menopause, and then it begins to subside. It is not a disease but a normal condition.

This lumpiness is caused by the cyclic hormonal stimulation of the breast during each menstrual cycle. If conception does not take place the cellular growth in the milk ducts regresses, and the excess blood and water that makes the breasts fuller during the pre-menstrual phase also subside. But before the breasts can fully return to their previous state, another menstrual cycle is well underway and the rising hormones again stimulate a proliferation of glandular tissue.

Some women are barely aware of these changes, but many experience considerable swelling and tenderness, especially during the pre-menstrual phase (see Figure 15). The symptoms tend to worsen with age, and, as some women approach menopause, they find that their breasts are almost constantly swollen and tender.

This subsides after menopause. However, post-menopausal women who take replacement hormones may continue to have fibrocystic breasts.

Women who have had the more routine fibrocystic tenderness for years should not be alarmed by this more chronic aspect. While it is true that there is a rise in the incidence of breast cancer at this time in a woman's life, she should rest assured that the fibrocystic lumpiness has nothing to do with the disease. However, it remains important for a woman in her late forties and early fifties to be particularly

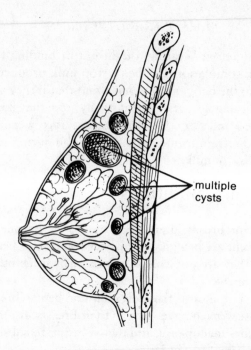

multiple
cysts

Figure 15. Cysts typical of a fibrocystic breast during pre-menstrual phase, when hormonal influences peak

diligent about breast self-examination and periodic examinations by her doctor.

Ultrasound, most associated with scans for pregnant women, also gives excellent 'pictures' of the breast and, combined with mammography, helps hospital doctors and radiologists to reach quite accurate diagnoses of breast problems.

Any discomfort can generally be relieved by a mild analgesic such as aspirin. Wearing a well-fitted bra that gives adequate support also helps. A larger size may be needed for the pre-menstrual period, and some women find that wearing a bra all the time, including in bed, is helpful. Cutting down on salt intake may help reduce fluid retention and swelling; if this is not sufficient, a diuretic may be prescribed.

Abstaining from products that contain methylxanthines – found in coffee, chocolate, tea, some soft drinks and medicines may help to prevent pre-menstrual breast tenderness. It has not been proved that methylxanthines cause breast tenderness. Still, enough women obtain relief to lead some doctors to recommend a trial period of avoiding food or beverages that contain them.

If these conservative measures are inadequate to relieve the breast symptoms, hormone treatment may help. The pill often helps breast symptoms subside or disappear. Tamoxifen, an anti-oestrogen drug, may reduce breast nodularity and relieve the swelling and pain. The cause may also be an underactive thyroid, and when treated, the breast symptoms may be relieved. Danazol may also relieve breast symptoms, but it carries a number of side effects, mentioned earlier, that limit its use for this purpose.

In extreme instances, a woman with fibrocystic lumpiness and large, difficult-to-examine breasts, may be subjected to repeated biopsies and this makes her very fearful of cancer. There have been instances in which women in this situation have undergone preventive mastectomies followed by breast reconstruction. Obviously, this is a serious undertaking and one that should be considered only as a last resort. The large majority of women who suffer from this extreme fibrocystic condition and cancer phobia can be helped by counselling, and certainly this should be undertaken before any surgery.

Breast cysts

Frequently a woman will develop a cyst that is not necessarily related to fibrocystic breasts. Cysts often appear suddenly – one day there is nothing, and the next a woman may be alarmed to discover a large lump. Typically, a cyst is round, smooth and firm, but can be compressed when squeezed. They are most common in the premenopausal years, but can develop at any age. Following ultrasound/mammography, as mentioned earlier, a cyst can be drained with a hollow needle; if it does not disappear with drainage or reappears in a few days, it should be further checked for possible cancer cells. But it may well be quicker for the two to be combined. The reason is that since the identification of different cells in the body has now become so routine with technological advances, a hospital pathology or histology lab can speed up the process. In addition, it may be the cells, not the fluid, which are directly causing the trouble. Cysts larger than 3mm are common and occur in some 7 per cent of all women. An increased risk of breast cancer is there but small, relating to only 2 to 4 per cent of those 7 per cent of women.

Fibroadenomas

Fibroadenomas are another relatively common benign breast condition that manifests itself with a lump. Usually rounded, firm and painless, they move freely when examined with the fingers. Normally, they appear singly, but sometimes a woman will develop several and in rare instance, there may be 20 or more fibroadenomas scattered throughout a woman's breast.

Typically a fibroadenoma first appears when a woman is in her late teens or early 20s, but there are many exceptions in which they develop later in life. There have been reports that women using the pill are more prone to develop fibroadenomas, but the connection between the two has not been proved.

Nipple discharge

All women have a small amount of nipple discharge, and most are not aware of this. It keeps the nipple ducts open. Women on the pill or post-menopausal oestrogen replacement often experience increased nipple discharge and this is normal. A yellow crusting, that appears to clog them, is no more than hardened discharge and is easily washed off. But you should not keep squeezing the nipple, because you will keep making it discharge!

The first point to remember is that abnormal nipple discharges should always be checked by a doctor. If a woman starts to produce breastmilk, though she is not pregnant and has not recently breastfed, it is usually caused by a hormonal imbalance or milk cyst. Such a discharge can also have blood in it. However, bloody discharges are usually caused by an intraductal papilloma – a benign wart-like growth in the lining of a milk duct. They can also be a warning sign of cancer.

Mastitis

Mastitis is an inflammation of the breast, occurring most often in women who are breastfeeding. It may be caused by an obstructed milk duct. More often than not abscesses, requiring drainage, sometimes form. The breast may be engorged, and the skin looks like orange peel (peau d'orange), the classic indicator of an abscess. The axillary lymph nodes in the armpit on the affected side may also be enlarged. This condition should not be confused with the characteristics of the rare, but highly lethal, inflammatory breast cancer, where there are similarities, so have the mastitis checked out as soon as possible.

Fibrosis

This is a gradual replacement of glandular breast tissue by inert, fibrous tissue. Typically, a woman will notice areas that feel firm and thickened, with indistinct boundaries. It may develop at the site of a previous infection or surgical scar, but more often, there is no apparent cause. Investigation should be done to make sure that it is, in fact, fibrosis and then no treatment is required.

Sclerosing adenosis

This is an overgrowth of glandular tissue, which eventually crowds out some of the normal connective tissue of the breast. The body tries to stop it by producing fibrous cells. It may be a mass or spread throughout the breast. Investigations will confirm that the tissue is not cancerous, and no further treatment is called for.

Fat necrosis

This is the death of fat cells, usually caused by an injury or inflammation; sometimes this occurs after rapid weight loss. It may also be related to natural breast changes that come with age. The dead cells eventually calcify and fibrous tissue may grow around them, forming a hard, irregular lump. Mammography usually can distinguish between the calcification of fat necrosis and the calcium deposits that accompany cancer. Full investigations are advised.

Nipple papillomas and polyps

Papillomas are wart-like growths in a milk-duct lining near the nipple. They usually produce a bloody discharge, and may be felt as a small lump. They are quite rare, usually only occurring in pre-menopausal women. A papilloma can generally be diagnosed by a microscopic study of the bloody discharge, but a surgical biopsy may be needed. They are not generally linked to cancer though some types may have a role in cancer.

Nipple polyps are small growths that form on the skin, often re-sembling tiny mushrooms, with a thin stalk and rounded head. They are harmless, but women often want to have them removed because

143

of their appearance or because they may become irritated if they rub against clothing and cause discomfort.

Breast cancer

Breast cancer is the most serious of all breast diseases. Unfortunately, it is also one the most common among women in industrialised countries and a leading killer.

At some time during their lives, one out of every 11 European women will develop breast cancer. Diagnosis and treatment of breast cancer have improved but the death rate has not really changed in 50 years. This is attributed to the fact that the disease strikes mostly older women, a group which is growing.

Although hormones appear to play a definite role in many breast cancers, the cause of the disease is unknown. Several factors that increase the risk of breast cancer have been identified and include previous breast cancer, a family history of the disease, a long menstrual history marked by early menarche and late menopause, and a high-fat, high-calorie diet. Women more than 20 per cent above ideal weight have a somewhat higher incidence of the disease, as do women whose first full-term pregnancy was after the age of 30.

These risk factors are by no means predictive or uniform. Many breast cancer specialists say all women must be considered to be at high risk, and therefore must be very diligent about breast self-examination and regular check-ups by a doctor even if they have no family history of the disease. Early diagnosis and treatment afford the best chance of surviving breast cancer. Up to 90 per cent or even more of all women whose cancer is detected and treated while it is still small and confined to the breast can be cured of the disease. That definition means being free of any evidence of cancer five years after treatment. This cure rate falls to less than 50 per cent if the cancer already has spread to the lymph nodes, a sign that malignant cells may already have travelled to other parts of the body.

About 90 per cent of all breast cancers are initially detected by the woman herself, which is why regular breast self-examination is so important. All women over the age of 20 should systematically examine their breasts each month. For women who are menstruating, this should be done a week to 10 days after the start of a period, when the breasts are smallest and easiest to examine. Post-menopausal women should mark their calendars to remind them to examine their breasts on the first day of each month. Despite the widespread publicity given to the need for regular breast self-examination far too few women do it.

Unfortunately many women, like many in Italy for example, mistakenly believe that breast self-examination is contrary to the dictates of the Catholic Church. Similarly, some women may shun breast self-examination as well as examination by a male doctor because they believe it may be immoral.

All women should have an annual breast examination, apart from any that they do themselves at home. There are now a number of women who either ask their doctor, or pay privately, for a mammography.

Do not let finding a lump in your breast make you lose your composure. Most breast lumps turn out to be benign. Fear must not cause you to delay seeing a doctor, because there is no point in worrying over a benign growth or allowing a fast-growing cancer cause risk of death. Any woman who finds a lump or other suspicious sign, such as dimpling of the skin, distortion, engorgement, or other change, *should see her doctor as soon as possible.*

The diagnostic procedure involves physical examination – often, a doctor can tell by a characteristic feel whether a lump is a harmless cyst or something that should be investigated further – and sometimes with mammography and a biopsy, which may be done either with an aspiration needle or surgically. A biopsy, which entails removing a small amount of tissue and examining it microscopically, is always needed for a definitive diagnosis of any suspicious lump. A biopsy is not needed if there is no doubt that a lump is a harmless cyst (a fact that can be confirmed by withdrawing its fluid), or a normal part of breast anatomy. Most biopsies can be done on an outpatient basis with a local anaesthetic. Exceptions include instances in which the mass is deep within the breast or is affixed to the chest wall, or when a suspicious area shows up in a mammogram but cannot be felt. The best course for the latter is to use mammography and special dyes to mark the suspicious area before having biopsy tissue removed.

There is another vital diagnostic test that is often done at the time of a biopsy of any suspected malignant tissue. This is a hormone-receptor assay to measure the sensitivity of the cancer to oestrogen and, to a lesser degree, progesterone. This must be done on fresh tissue at the time of the biopsy. The results may not necessarily alter the initial course of treatment, but are important if the cancer recurs or if there is evidence of spread. If the cancer recurs, the hormone-receptor tests would be repeated because the new cancers are not always of the same cellular type as the original one.

Hormones and breast cancer

The precise role of hormones in breast cancer is not fully understood, but it appears that the growth of some cancers is stimulated by the female sex hormones. Researchers think that this may explain why obese women have a higher incidence of breast cancer than normal-weight women – the fat cells convert adrenal hormones to oestrogen, and this high level of oestrogen is thought to stimulate growth of hormone-dependent cancers. Also, overweight women are likely to have high cholesterol levels, which may increase breast-cancer risk.

Hormone manipulation in the treatment of breast cancer is now more precisely targeted to those women most likely to benefit and it can help perhaps a third of women with advanced breast cancer.

The concept behind hormone therapy for breast cancer originated in the late 1880s with observations that removal of the ovaries of a woman with breast cancer could cause the tumour to shrink. A half-century later, researchers set about trying to refine this approach. In a study that began in 1948, several hundred pre-menopausal women with breast cancer agreed to undergo radical mastectomies, followed by radiation to their ovaries to make them stop producing hormones. The women who underwent this premature, artificial menopause lived longer, without recurrence of cancer, than women who were treated with mastectomies alone.

At about the same time, other researchers observed that some women who received oestrogen also experienced shrinking of their breast cancers – a seeming contradiction to the other findings. These early studies indicated that younger women who were still menstruating, were the most likely to benefit from inducing an artificial menopause, while older, post-menopausal women were most likely to respond to additive hormone therapy. But not all women in either group benefited from these strategies, and with the development of anti-cancer drugs in the 1960s, chemotherapy gained favour over hormonal manipulation in the treatment of advanced breast cancer.

Today, thanks to hormone-receptor tests which help identify women who are most likely to be helped by this therapy, hormonal manipulation is again a mainstay of breast-cancer treatment. Researchers have found that about two out of three women will have positive hormone receptors, indicating that their cancers are stimulated by oestrogen, progesterone or both.

Pre-menopausal women are less likely to have oestrogen-dependent cancers than older women who have gone through menopause. Among women whose cancers have recurred or spread to other parts of the body, about half of these will improve with some sort of hormonal manipulation. The higher the level of receptors, the more likely a woman is to benefit from hormone treatment.

The form of hormonal therapy depends upon a woman's age and whether she has gone through menopause. Pre-menopausal women are likely to receive some sort of removal treatment to reduce the amount of circulating oestrogen. At one time, this usually meant removing the ovaries surgically or damaging them with radiation treatment to halt their hormone production. Today, a woman is more likely to take an anti-oestrogen drug, usually tamoxifen, which results in a chemical menopause.

Other possible hormonal treatments include taking a drug called aminoglutethimide to block the adrenal glands from producing steroid hormones. The objective is to rid the body of androstenedione, which is secreted by the adrenal glands and converted by fat cells into a form of oestrogen.

Although this is not the practice in the UK, there is another procedure – the surgical removal of the adrenal glands. After this operation, the woman will have to take hydrocortisone to replace that which is normally made by the adrenal glands. Similarly, but not usually in the UK, in some instances, the pituitary gland may be removed to rid the body of prolactin, which may stimulate the growth of some breast cancers. The woman then must take replacement hormones to maintain proper fluid and salt balance.

In the past, male sex hormones were given to women with advanced breast cancer, a strategy that produced remission in about 15 per cent of women who were pre-menopausal or who had only recently gone through menopause. However, these hormones produced severe side effects in women, including pronounced hairiness and virilisation, and their use has been replaced by tamoxifen.

Sometimes the use of progestogen produces improvement in women with advanced breast cancer but why, and how, is not known; it is usually given with oestrogen following the failure of anti-oestrogen drugs. Steroids with anti-cancer drugs do not appear to alter advanced metastatic cancer itself, but may relieve symptoms of metastases to the lungs, brain and bones.

Hormonal manipulation may be combined with cancer chemo-therapy, especially for a fast-growing tumour such as in inflammatory cancer. It takes about four months to achieve a remis-sion with hormonal manipulation, whereas cancer chemotherapy produces much faster results. Therefore, three or more chemother-apy agents are usually given immediately to initiate a regression.

Mastectomy – still the leading treatment

Although hormone manipulation is an important facet of treating breast cancer, mastectomy remains the most common and most effective treatment. Regrettably enormous numbers of total mastec-tomies were done, mainly by male surgeons, which were unnecessary and very traumatic. But in the last decade, the medical community has greatly revised its thinking regarding the extent of surgery needed to give a woman her best chance of overcoming breast cancer. The Halsted radical mastectomy, named after the pioneering surgeon who developed it in 1882, was the favoured operation. This procedure entails removal of the entire breast as well as the underlying chest muscle and the axillary lymph nodes from the adjacent armpit. The operation produces considerable deformity. It reduced the very high mortality rate that prevailed before its inception but it was not until 1948, and much later in general usage, that it was shown to be often unnecessary.

It was in 1948 that a British surgeon, D. H. Patey, developed the modified radical mastectomy, in which he removed the breast and axillary nodes, but left the underlying chest muscle in place. Studies demonstrated that this operation lowered recurrence and mortality just as much as the classic Halsted procedure, but it did not produce as much chest deformity. It has also taken too long for surgeons to sufficiently recognise that in instances of small, localised cancer, removal of the lump (lumpectomy), followed by radiation therapy can be just as effective as a mastectomy.

A lack of informed consent, combined with the taboos and silence surrounding breast cancer have cost many women dear. This has happened in cases where surgeons, performing what should only have been an exploratory biopsy, have carried out a radical mastectomy, if they found a cancerous growth, while the woman was under anaesthetic. This controversy within the medical community has coincided with the growing awareness among women that they should have more control over their bodies.

Such instances have undoubtedly caused many women to delay treatment for a suspicious breast lump. The treatment was as dreaded as the disease itself. The surgeon's primary concern was in saving the woman's life, and little attention was paid to the emotional consequences.

This has now changed dramatically but you need to make sure that you ask fully and get full answers about any surgery recommended for your condition. Women now have more say in their treatment decisions, and doctors should be more sensitive to the emotional aspects of breast cancer for both the woman and her family. The most common operation is now the modified radical mastectomy, increasingly followed by breast reconstruction to overcome the deformity of losing a breast.

For small (less than 4cm/1½in) cancers that are confined to the breast, a lumpectomy or partial mastectomy followed by radiation therapy may be just as effective as more extensive surgery. In this procedure, the cancer and a small amount of surrounding cancer-free tissue are removed and the axillary lymph nodes are dissected for evidence of spread. As soon as the wound has healed sufficiently, a woman will begin radiation therapy, which is aimed at killing any cancer cells that may have been missed in the operation.

Many breast specialists are still sceptical that this approach will produce as great a chance of a cure as a modified radical mastectomy, but several studies suggest that it may be just as effective.

Even though many breast surgeons do not favour a partial mastectomy, most now agree that a woman should be more informed and allowed to participate in the decision-making process. The former one-step biopsy/treatment procedure is now seldom done, and if it is, a tentative diagnosis of cancer will have been made before the operation. In this situation a woman will be given an opportunity to get a second opinion and explore other treatment options. Some women may not want to participate in the decision-making process, but increasingly, they are the exceptions and not the norm as in the past. Second opinions are your right and you should also ask to meet with a plastic surgeon before a mastectomy to plan breast reconstruction. If you encounter pressure not to be properly involved, seek advice about going elsewere and do not delay.

Obviously, breast cancer is still a difficult disease, but today's approach makes it easier for both the woman and her family to cope with its consequences. Improved reconstruction techniques make it easier for a woman to accept the loss of a breast. Although there is no cure yet for breast cancer once it has spread beyond the breast, increasing numbers of women are enjoying many years of comfortable, productive life thanks to combinations of treatments that can create remissions. And today's increased emphasis on early diagnosis and treatment is paying off in improved chances of a cure.

Summing up

A woman's breasts are more than milk-producing glands; they also are objects of sexual attraction and, to many, the embodiment of femininity and maternal nurturing. Breasts are particularly sensitive to hormonal changes, and many breast disorders are hormone-related. Breast cancer remains one of the most common and serious of all breast diseases. All women must be attuned to the early warning signs of breast cancer and seek prompt treatment, thereby giving themselves their best chance of overcoming this most dangerous of all female cancers.

CHAPTER NINE

Ovarian Disorders

The ovaries, the small, egg-shaped glands tucked deep within the pelvic cavity are, in a real sense a woman's 'key' glands. One on each side of the uterus, and close to the fallopian tubes, they are formed about four weeks after conception takes place. By the fifth month of gestation, the foetal ovaries contain six to seven million immature egg follicles. No new follicles are ever formed; their number declines to about two million by the time of birth. During the reproductive years, only 300–500 of these follicles develop into mature eggs. The others wither and die.

A girl's ovaries are quiescent, producing only a very small amount of hormones until puberty. As puberty approaches, the ovaries 'wake up', because of the stimulation of the pituitary's gonadotropin hormones. As the ovaries increase their output of oestrogen, the girl develops the secondary female characteristics – breasts, pubic and axillary hair and the rounded curves of a woman's figure. The onset of menstruation is the culmination of this development.

Each month, during a woman's reproductive years one, and sometimes more, of the egg follicles ripens and is released ready for fertilisation. This is ovulation, controlled by a complex, finely-tuned hormonal feedback system.

The ovaries are exquisitely sensitive to what is going on elsewhere in the body, so scores of factors can interfere with their function. If a woman is under- or overweight, if the thyroid fails to produce the proper amount of hormones, or if she is ill, the ovaries may shut down. This is actually a protective sensitivity – it ensures that, should conception take place the developing foetus will have the best

151

environment. Of course, the system is not foolproof: there are times when conception takes place under extremely adverse conditions and times when the ovaries fail to function for no apparent reason.

After regular ovulation is established, usually one to two years after menarche, a woman can expect to have an average of 13 cycles of 28–29 days each every year. The length of the cycles varies, but between 21–35 days is considered normal. In addition, all women occasionally have cycles in which they bleed but do not ovulate. Among younger women this may happen only once or twice a year, but as a woman grows older, the number of anovulatory cycles increases.

During the first, or follicular phase of the menstrual cycle, there is a steady rise in follicle-stimulating hormone prompting the ovary to prepare a follicle to mature. This causes a steady rise in oestrogen during the follicular phase, with a rapid increase as the follicle nears maturity. There is then a brief decline which signals the hypothalamus to tell the pituitary to increase production of LH and FSH. The surge in these gonadotrophins raises the oestrogen level again. Up to this point the level of circulating progesterone has been very low; just before ovulation the follicle begins to increase progesterone production, and blood levels of the hormone rise sharply. Other hormones, including prolactin and growth hormone also rise during this mid-cycle period.

The surge of FSH and LH prompts release of the mature egg from the follicle that then develops into the corpus luteum, a term for the yellowish fat of its structure. The corpus luteum secretes large amounts of progesterone, the hormone that prepares the endometrium for the fertilised egg and maintains pregnancy after conception. If the egg is not fertilised by the time it reaches the uterus – a journey of four to six days – there is a sharp drop in progesterone and oestrogen and the endometrium begins to break down. Fourteen days after ovulation, menstruation (the shedding of the uterine lining) takes place. Prostaglandins secreted by the uterus are thought to help facilitate menstruation by causing contractions of the uterine muscles. Excessive prostaglandins are believed to be responsible for the cramps many women experience in the first two days of their period.

The hormonal changes during menstruation are responsible for varied physical and emotional changes. Pre-menstrual tension has already been discussed in Chapter 4. Many women feel an increase in sexual desire at about mid-cycle – believed to be due to rise in androgens. It is known that the androgens are involved in shaping female libido. (They also control male libido, but in men the testes are the major source of the hormones.) The role of oestrogen in sexual desire is unknown. Taking extra oestrogen does not increase libido in a normal healthy woman, but removing the ovaries will lower sexual drive, while giving replacement oestrogen will revive it.

During the pre-menstrual phase, many women experience diminished interest in sex, but the reason for this is not known. Contrary to popular belief, orgasm and the ability to achieve it is not controlled by hormones; it is an involuntary reflex during which there is a sudden release of muscular tension and congested blood vessels produced by sexual stimulation. Women of all ages are capable of orgasm, regardless of their hormonal status. In fact, many older women find that they are more sexually responsive and achieve orgasm easier than when they were younger. The reasons for this are probably both psychological and physical.

Amenorrhoea

The failure to menstruate is called amenorrhoea and arises because the ovaries do not work properly. The ovaries, of course are highly sensitive and are affected by almost all the other endocrine glands. Thus any hormonal imbalance can result in amenorrhoea. Most often amenorrhoea is not associated with any disorder – undetected pregnancy is one of the most common causes. Menopause, both natural and artificial, is another. Other causes include emotional stress, use of the contraceptive pill and other drugs and weight loss (due to anorexia nervosa or rigorous exercise). Other reasons could be diabetes and other illnesses, tumours, infection, ovarian cysts and other conditions that have already been discussed in Chapter 4.

It is generally acceptable to wait until a girl is 16 before becoming concerned about primary amenorrhoea or the failure to start menstruating. However if there are other signs of abnormalities, such as the lack of sexual development, then there is need for concern. Primary amenorrhoea is relatively rare; in 60 per cent of cases it can be attributed to congenital defects that affect ovarian or genital development. The remaining 40 per cent can be traced to hormonal disorders, cystic ovaries and ovarian or uterine disorders.

The doctor will usually review medical history with special reference to growth and development during puberty. If it appears that development of sexual characteristics has been normal it is a sign that the ovaries have functioned and that the problem may lie in a structural abnormality. This is known as testicular feminisation. If a young woman has normal breasts, but no pubic or axillary hair, the problem may be caused by a chromosomal abnormality in which a person develops female characteristics, but has a male genetic makeup.

There is a relatively common condition in which women have irregular periods, have excess growth of hair and become infertile. This is called the adrenogenital syndrome or congenital adrenal-hyperplasia and requires hormonal treatment.

Chromosomal abnormalities

All body cells with nuclei have 46 chromosomes. The exceptions are the egg and the sperm which have 23 each to make a total of 46 when they unite. The female genotype carries two X (female) sex chromosomes, while the male genotype has an X and a Y (male) chromosome. Thus the female egg always carries the X or female characteristic, while the sperm may carry either male or female characteristics. If an egg is fertilised with a Y chromosome, the baby will be a boy; an X sperm will produce a girl. The Y chromosome carries a gene that controls formation of testes in the embryo. These embryonic testes secrete hormones that further develop the male reproductive tract.

In rare instances, something goes amiss at the moment of conception. For example, an abnormal sperm that lacks the X or Y chromosome may fertilise an egg; instead of an XX genotype, the baby will have an XO. Similarly, an XO genotype can be produced by a normal X sperm fertilising an egg lacking an X chromosome. (An X chromosome is needed to produce a viable foetus; there are no recorded instances of a YO foetus, which would have only the male genotype, surviving.) Since an XX genotype is required to form normal ovaries, babies born without this combination (they would have an XO structure) may have female characteristics, but will lack properly functioning ovaries. A person with an XO genotype (about one of every 2,500 females) is known as having Turner's syndrome.

A woman with Turner's syndrome may be short, have a thick webbed neck, underdeveloped breasts and immature genitals. The ovaries are absent being replaced by streaks of tissue. A number of other congenital abnormalities may accompany Turner's syndrome. These could be auto-immune disease, thyroid disorder, diabetes, hearing loss, possible increased susceptibility to some types of cancer, growth disorders and kidney abnormalities.

Sometimes the defect may be apparent at an early age, but usually it does not become evident till puberty. A girl with Turner's syndrome will develop breasts but sparse pubic and axillary hair. Oestrogen therapy is started during adolescence but care should be taken not to give it too early as it will further diminish growth. With oestrogen therapy the girl will develop normal female secondary sex characteristics. If she has a normal uterus, she will menstruate if she is also given progesterone.

In the past women with Turner's syndrome have been hopelessly infertile, even though they may have a normal uterus. Recent advances in in-vitro fertilisation and embryo transplants now make it possible for some of these women to become mothers by obtaining donor eggs that are fertilised by their husband's sperm and then transferred to their own uterus. But such women will need to have proper hormonal therapy to support a pregnancy.

Very occasionally a baby is born with poorly differentiated sexual characteristics. In very rare cases the baby may be a hermaphrodite, with both ovarian and testicular tissue. The external genitals may be mixed, but male characteristics usually dominate. This sexual ambiguity is usually treated surgically, by removing the less dominant sexual characteristics.

It is more common for a baby to be a pseudo-hermaphrodite. This means it will have different external genitalia and internal reproductive organs. In order for the male embryo to develop the right reproductive organs for its sex, its testes must produce the right hormones during the embryonic stage. Until about the eighth week of gestation, the gonads of males and females are indistinguishable, and, without male hormones, they will develop into female reproductive organs regardless of genotype. If the male embryo has androgen insensitivity – the hormones are present in normal amounts but the peripheral tissue cannot respond because of a receptor abnormality – then it will develop testicular feminisation. The baby will be born with testes (often hidden inside the body) and female external genitalia (a vagina, but no uterus or fallopian tubes). These children are generally reared as girls; with puberty, breasts may develop, but with little or no sexual hair. Fortunately, this is a rare condition.

If the testes are removed before puberty, oestrogen and progestogen therapy should be given to stimulate breast and secondary sex hair development. Women with these chromosomal abnormalities are infertile, and there is no treatment that can correct the condition. They usually have a vaginal canal, however, and can have normal sexual relations.

Occasionally the use of hormone preparations during the first three months of pregnancy can cause sexual abnormalities in the foetus. Progestogens used to be given to women to prevent miscarriage; nearly three per cent of girls born to these women had some degree of masculinisation of their external genitalia. Danazol (a drug derived from testosterone) is used to treat endometriosis; it has sometimes been taken by women who did not realise they were pregnant, resulting in girls being born with male genitalia. Large amounts of stilboestrol, a synthetic oestrogen, that was also once prescribed to prevent miscarriage, also can cause masculinisation.

In unusual cases, a mother may have a tumour that produces male hormones. These not only cause virilisation in the woman but can also result in the masculinisation of a female foetus should the tumour be present in early pregnancy. Although this may be very distressing for the parents, the situation is easily rectified. The effects are usually confined to external genitalia, and these can be surgically corrected at the appropriate time. The girls are generally born with proper internal reproductive organs; with puberty they will develop into normal women.

It is important that hormonal drugs be avoided if there is any chance that a woman may be pregnant or that conception may take place while they are being used.

Ovarian cysts

Multiple cysts in the ovaries are one of the more common causes of menstrual irregularities and failure to ovulate. They are difficult to remove surgically because they are extremely small, sometimes smaller than a ripe follicle before it is liberated, though others may be considerably larger.

What initiates this syndrome is unknown, but once it is set in motion, it perpetuates itself, with increasing hormonal imbalances. In normal circumstances the rise of oestrogen in the first phase of the menstrual cycle triggers the pituitary to increase secretion of FSH and LH. In response to these gonad-stimulating hormones, one or more ovarian follicles begin to mature. One or two of them grow faster than the others, reaching up to three-quarters of an inch in diameter.

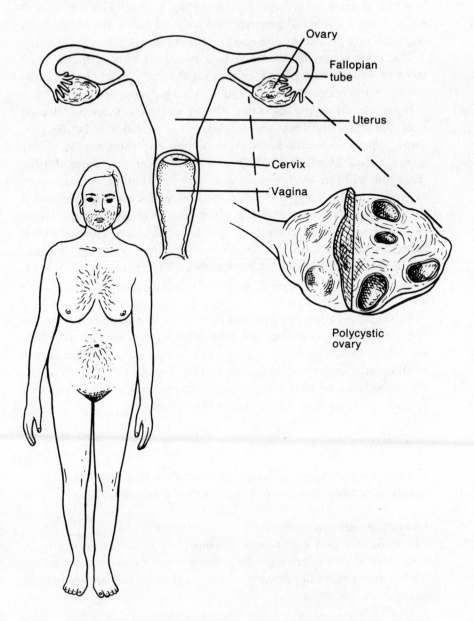

Figure 16. Changes that accompany polycystic ovary: there may be signs of virilisation, such as increased hairiness on face, chest and abdomen

157

When the egg matures, it bursts from the sac and the large follicle in which it grew is replaced by the corpus luteum. This begins secreting large amounts of progesterone to build and maintain the lush uterine lining primed by the earlier surge of oestrogen.

The cysts generally disappear in a month or two, without treatment. A woman may not be aware that she had a cyst, but for some the condition becomes chronic and is called polycystic ovaries.

In this condition the egg is not released in mid-cycle, being released later. Menstruation becomes irregular – the period may be delayed, come every two weeks for a cycle or two and then not occur for several cycles. Bleeding may be heavier than usual – a feature of menstruation without ovulation. There may be abdominal pain from expanding cysts. The ovaries become enlarged with white cysts and thickened thecal cells. Ovarian physiology is disturbed and more male hormones than normal are produced. The egg cannot escape from the thickened thecal walls, so ovulation does not occur. Because of the large amounts of androgens being secreted, a woman with polycystic ovaries often will become hairier than normal and may also be troubled by acne.

Polycystic ovarian changes can be treated by taking hormones to stimulate ovulation. In the past, part of the ovaries were removed by surgery – ovarian wedge re-section. This is very rare today because it often created complications, such as adhesions in the abdomen. On the other hand, modern drug therapy, though not 100 per cent successful, is much better and has fewer side effects.

Tumours

There are a number of relatively rare tumours that produce male or female hormones that interfere with normal ovulation.

Granulosa-theca cell tumours
The most common symptoms are related to excessive oestrogens. In some women there are signs of virilism from excessive androgens. The tumours generally develop after the age of 30 and between 10–20 per cent are malignant.

Androblastomas
Quite rare, the symptoms are related to virilism caused by excessive androgens. They occur in women between 20 and 40 years old.

Lipid cell tumours

There are two categories: one that produces oestrogens and the other, androgens. The former has a 20 per cent risk of malignancy; it is often associated with diabetes and seen in women between the ages of 20–50 years. The latter is rarely malignant and generally develops after the age of 45.

Ovarian cancer

Cancer of the ovaries is the third most common gynaecological cancer (preceded by cancers of the cervix and uterus/endometrium). The high death rate is due to the fact that the disease is not detected until a late stage. Unfortunately, a cervical smear which is very helpful in spotting the early stages of cervical cancer, is of no help as far as ovarian cancer is concerned. Studies are going on to see if ultrasound examination, a relatively simple procedure, will be able to pick up early signs of ovarian cancer.

The most common symptoms are abdominal swelling and discomfort, nausea, urinary urgency or retention, constipation and other gastro-intestinal problems that are caused by rapidly expanding growth and retention of fluid.

Should the doctor feel an ovarian growth during a pelvic examination, he may have a biopsy done, particularly if the woman is past menopause, which is the time when ovarian cancer is most common. However ultrasound first is the preferable option and then, if necessary, a laparoscopy can be done. The laparoscope is a viewing device that is inserted through an incision just below the navel.

About 85 per cent of ovarian cancers arise in the epithelial tissue that covers the ovaries. The rest originate in other types of cells. The ovaries are also susceptible to cancers that have spread from other parts of the body.

The role of hormones in causing ovarian cancer is not clear. Some studies have reported a somewhat higher incidence of this disease among post-menopausal women who take oestrogen. The ovary has oestrogen receptors, but these are not found in the epithelium (where most cancers originate). The cancers themselves have been found to contain receptors for both oestrogen and progesterone, and the use of progesterone has produced response rates of up to 38 per cent in some studies, but this is not a universal finding.

There are varying opinions on the risk of developing ovarian cancer. Some studies have found that women who have had several children are less likely to develop it, than those who are childless or who have had small families. Other researchers maintain that women who have been on the pill have a lower incidence of ovarian cancer. The exact causes are still not clear. The treatment is to remove the ovaries and other reproductive organs. If the cancer has spread to surrounding tissue, this too will be removed, if possible. Surgery may be followed by radiation therapy, and depending on the type of cancer, chemotherapy. However these do not always prevent recurrence of the cancer.

Hysterectomy

Removal of the ovaries need not necessarily be part of the hysterectomy operation. In the USA however, this has been quite common – millions of women have had this operation and for women over 40 it has often included removal of the ovaries. In the UK the Office of Population Censuses and Surveys says that 66,000 women have hysterectomies each year.

Removal of the ovaries creates an abrupt menopause that is invariably accompanied by hot flushes, mood swings and other menopausal symptoms. The body is not allowed to adjust to the tapering off of hormones, so the symptoms are frequently more severe than those in the natural menopause.

There have to be sound medical reasons for removal of the ovaries and increasingly women undergoing a hysterectomy are demanding that their ovaries are left intact. Practice in the UK now is generally to be cautious. Cancer elsewhere in the female reproductive tract often spreads to the ovaries and this is justification for their removal. But there is no reason to remove the ovaries of a woman who is having a hysterectomy due to benign fibroids or other such conditions. Studies have found that women who have their ovaries removed at an early age are much more likely to develop severe osteoporosis than women who enter a later, natural menopause. Ask for a second opinion on such removal if the hysterectomy is for a benign condition.

There are now hysterectomy support groups that help women. To find out if there if there is an HSG in your area, get in touch with your local Well Woman centre or its equivalent, or your local library will help find it for you.

Summing up

The ovaries are the woman's major source of sex hormones, and are also essential for normal reproductive function. These glands are extraordinarily sensitive to their environment and a large number of factors can affect their function. Some of these factors are relatively easy to identify. In other cases detailed detective work has to be done to locate the cause of ovarian failure. Recent advances in in-vitro fertilisation and embryo transfers now make it possible for women without ovaries, but with normal uteruses, to experience pregnancy and childbirth.

CHAPTER TEN

Diabetes and Hypoglycaemia

Diabetes, a chronic disease marked by the body's inability to properly metabolise carbohydrates and other foods, is the most common endocrine disorder in the world. There are quite often large numbers of sufferers who are undiagnosed and in the UK, for example, these are put at 500,000. In a UK population of about 57 million there are 750,000 diagnosed diabetics, a third of whom are insulin-dependent.

Over the last decade, our knowledge of how to control diabetes has progressed remarkably, and with proper management, today's diabetic patient can lead a normal, productive life. However, this requires a thorough knowledge of the disease and diligent attention to virtually every detail of living. A person with diabetes must monitor day-to-day activities that most of us never give a second thought to: diet, exercise, infection, stress, the menstrual cycle and dozens of factors can alter blood sugar and make diabetes worse.

There are two different forms of diabetes. In one, which has at least three names – Type 1, juvenile-onset, or insulin-dependent diabetes – the pancreas ceases to produce insulin. This is the hormone the body needs for a number of functions, especially utilisation of blood sugar (glucose), its major fuel. This type of diabetes requires daily injections of insulin and close attention to balancing the intake of fat, protein and carbohydrate. The insulin itself may be from animal extract or synthetic human insulin.

In the other form, which is known as Type 2, adult-onset or non-insulin-dependent diabetes, the pancreas may produce inadequate amounts of insulin. Sometimes the body is unable to make proper use

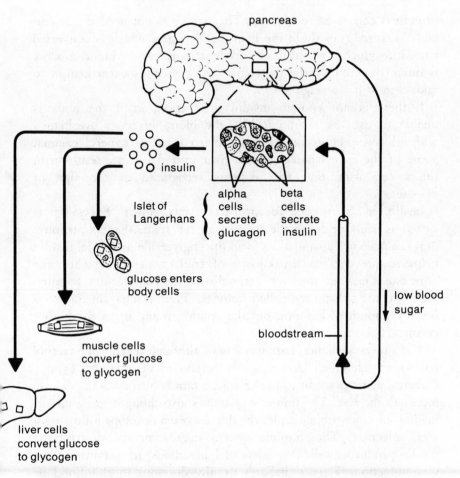

Figure 17. Insulin metabolism: low blood sugar inhibits the se-cretion of insulin; high blood sugar stimulates its secretion

of the insulin that is produced. Type 2 diabetes can often be treated by weight loss and exercise. Though it is a serious disease, it is not as life-threatening as uncontrolled Type 1 diabetes. Before the discovery of insulin in 1921, a person with Type 1 diabetes usually succumbed to it within a year or two.

Roles of insulin

Insulin is needed to regulate the amount of glucose that circulates in the blood. Almost all carbohydrate and 50 to 60 per cent of protein is converted to glucose. That which is not needed immediately is stored, mostly in the liver, as glycogen, which is converted back into glucose as the body needs it. Any rise in blood glucose is quickly sensed by the pancreas, which secretes extra insulin to take care of it (see Figure 17).

If there is not enough insulin production, or if the body is unable to use the insulin it has, the blood becomes overloaded with glucose. This condition is referred to as hyperglycaemia. Some of the excess glucose spills over into the urine, resulting in the sweet urine that the ancients recognised as the sign of diabetes.

Insulin is also needed for proper fat metabolism. Excess fat is stored as triglycerides in the adipose, or fat, tissue. Excess carbohydrate calories are also used to form the triglyceride molecule. Insulin helps to prevent the breakdown of triglycerides. But when the hormone is lacking, the liver metabolises these triglycerides, forming highly acidic substances called ketones. The muscles can utilise a certain amount of ketones, but they build up and upset the body's chemical balance.

The causes of diabetes are unknown, although several risk factors have been identified that make a person vulnerable. In Type 1 diabetes, genetics seems to play a role; a family history of the disease increases the risk. The immune system is also thought to be instrumental. In susceptible people, the disease often develops following a viral infection. The immune system may somehow destroy the insulin-producing cells (the Islets of Langerhans) in response to the viral infection. Type 1 diabetes usually develops in childhood or young adulthood.

In Type 2 diabetes, the pancreas may produce insulin in varying amounts. In fact, some patients have higher-than-normal levels of insulin, while others have sharply reduced insulin production. Most are middle-aged or older, and the majority are overweight. The extra weight may make a person more resistant to insulin, or may increase the body's need for the hormone.

Pregnancy can precipitate diabetes; about two to six per cent of all pregnant women develop gestational diabetes. It appears during pregnancy and disappears with childbirth. It is particularly serious for the foetus and is a major cause of stillbirths or death shortly after birth. These women are also more likely to develop diabetes late in life.

Signs of diabetes

The most common early symptoms of diabetes are insatiable thirst accompanied by copious urination, hunger, weight loss and weakness. Mood swings are common. People with diabetes are more susceptible to infections. For many women, one of the first signs is an increased vulnerability to vaginal infections. Male impotence also is common in diabetes.

Diabetes affects virtually every organ system in the body. Leg cramps or pins-and-needles resulting from nerve damage may occur. The disease may also cause eye problems and kidney damage. High blood pressure, elevated cholesterol and atherosclerosis (hardening of the arteries from fatty plaque) are all made worse by diabetes, but these are usually later effects of the disease.

The self-care concept

The concept of diabetes self-care has evolved well and has shown how patients can often look after their health better than health professionals. It has meant new freedom and greater control, not only of their disease but also over their lives, for many people with the Type 1 form. Of course, self-care has always been an important part of diabetes treatment, since it is the patient who has to learn to inject insulin and be alert to symptoms that indicate blood glucose is too low or too high.

In the past, this meant testing urine at least daily for the presence of sugar (glycosuria). Although urine tests provide useful information about diabetes control, they do not necessarily reflect the immediate picture, and consequently, do not tell a patient what he or she should do at that moment to correct any imbalance. This shortcoming has been remedied by the development of new blood tests that enable a person to measure his or her own blood glucose within a minute or two, and take whatever action is appropriate to normalise sugar levels. By keeping careful daily records of blood sugar levels, food and insulin intake, exercise and other factors that affect the body's metabolism, a diabetic patient can avoid dangerous swings in blood glucose, and, most experts agree, prevent many of the serious complications of diabetes.

Successful diabetes self-care requires balancing the amount of insulin that is injected with the intake of food. Exercise and other circumstances that affect the body's uptake of insulin also must be taken into consideration. For example, a person who engages in regular vigorous exercise will not need as many units of insulin as a more sedentary person. A diabetic woman may require extra insulin during the pre-menstrual phase of her monthly cycle to overcome the anti-insulin affects of the female hormones that are high at that time. Stress and infection also make blood glucose more difficult to control.

After diabetes has been diagnosed by blood tests it is important that the patient learns how to measure his or her blood sugar and get a balance. This may involve intensive education sessions. At first, some people have difficulty giving themselves insulin injections or pricking a finger to draw the drop or two of blood that is needed to measure glucose levels. But the large majority of people find that, in a week or two, they have mastered not only the injection routine, but that they also can measure blood glucose in a couple of minutes. A variety of automated glucose meters are now widely available that help to remove much of the guesswork from measuring blood sugars.

Type 2 diabetes may be best managed with a diet and exercise programme, or an oral drug to stimulate insulin secretion and uptake may be prescribed if these conservative measures are not effective. The medication helps the glucose to be metabolised and thus overcome the 'barrier' or insulin-resistance which characterises Type 2 diabetes.

Diabetics need to pay special attention to keeping their toenails trimmed and groomed to avoid developing ingrowing toenails. These can lead to serious foot infections, especially if circulation to the lower limbs is impaired.

The pregnant diabetic

Self-care is particularly important for a diabetic woman who wants to have a baby. Only a few years ago, a pregnant woman with diabetes faced very discouraging odds for both herself and the baby.

A woman's chances of having a healthy baby increase if she can keep her blood glucose in the normal range throughout pregnancy. To achieve this, a woman must be extraordinarily motivated and attuned to her body. She also must know how to adjust her insulin dosage to meet her changing needs. She should discuss her plans with both the doctor who treats her diabetes and liaise with her local midwife and hospital maternity unit. Since pregnancy often extends some of the more common complications of diabetes – especially eye and kidney problems, high blood pressure and heart disease – extra caution must be exercised by a woman who already has any of these.

Pregnancy has profound effects on diabetes and the body's need for and utilisation of insulin. The placenta manufactures anti-insulin hormones and enzymes and the high levels of oestrogen and progesterone during pregnancy alter carbohydrate metabolism. If a woman's levels of blood glucose are too high, the foetus will respond by increasing its own insulin production. Since insulin acts as a foetal growth hormone, this can result in an oversized baby. These big babies are likely to be very sick at birth, and those who survive often have serious birth defects. Maintaining a normal blood glucose level throughout pregnancy can prevent excess foetal growth and the other congenital abnormalities associated with diabetes.

For several months before a diabetic woman attempts pregnancy, she should make sure that her blood sugar levels are normal and that other possible complications such as high blood pressure, are under good control. If she is not already keeping daily blood glucose charts, she should do so. While this kind of meticulous record-keeping may seem like a lot of bother at first, it is important for both the woman and her doctor because it provides a day-to-day overview as to the state of the diabetes as well as a basis for corrective steps.

During pregnancy, a woman should plan to measure her blood glucose six to eight times a day: upon rising, before and after meals and at bedtime. She should know how to adjust her food and insulin dosage to keep her blood glucose normal. It is particularly important that a pregnant diabetic woman eat on a regular schedule. Typically, this means three meals and three or four snacks a day, but some women may need to eat even more often, depending on the blood sugar levels and their symptoms.

Diligent self-monitoring and constant adjustment of insulin, food and exercise are so important during pregnancy. Diabetic mothers universally agree that the outcome – a normal, healthy baby – is worth the considerable effort.

Gestational diabetes

Two to 6 per cent of pregnant women develop a temporary type of diabetes that disappears almost immediately after delivery. In the past this often went undiagnosed and was the leading cause of late foetal death and stillbirths. Today it should be routinely tested for and diagnosed; the woman must monitor her blood sugar and take insulin as though she had regular Type 1 diabetes.

Women who are at a high risk for gestational diabetes should be tested more often, for example, at weeks 12, 18, and 32. Some of the risk factors include obesity, a family history of diabetes, a history of sugar in the urine, glucose intolerance or previous gestational diabetes, personal birthweight of more than 4kg (nine pounds), and recurrent urinary infections during pregnancy. Previous miscarriages, stillbirths, large babies, toxaemia, excessive amniotic fluid, or congenital defects, also indicate an increased risk of gestational diabetes (see Chapter 5).

At one time, doctors were reluctant to let a diabetic woman proceed to full term for a natural labour and delivery – an understandable caution given the large number of late foetal deaths and stillbirths. With the development of self-monitoring and improved blood glucose control, more obstetricians are now willing to let a pregnant diabetic go to full term and normal delivery. But from 34 weeks she will be asked to be particularly attuned to foetal movements. Any drop in kicking and other activity is a warning sign to call the doctor immediately. A drop in insulin requirements or other changes also warrant immediate investigation. During the last few weeks before delivery, the doctor also may want to check the baby's heart rate more often.

If there are any signs of foetal distress, tests may be done to assess the baby's status and its degree of maturity. If the baby's lungs are fully developed, many doctors will go ahead and induce labour or do a Caesarean section on the theory that, by this time, the baby will probably be better off on the outside. As soon as the baby is full-term, most obstetricians would prefer to induce labour if it does not start on its own, More commonly, however, if a woman has managed to keep her diabetes in good control throughout her pregnancy, she is likely to have a normal labour and delivery.

Reactive hypoglycaemia

Periodically the popular media 'discover' a new disease, often with vague, troubling symptoms that most people experience from time to time, for which doctors can find no cause.

Hypoglycaemia is the medical term for low blood sugar, or glucose, and it can occur in diabetes and other conditions when the amount of insulin circulating in the blood is more than is needed to metabolise available sugar. In diabetics it occurs most often when too much insulin has been injected, resulting in a rapid depletion of available blood glucose. Signs of this kind of insulin reaction include tingling sensations, particularly in the mouth and fingers, buzzing in the ears, a cold, clammy feeling, pallor, excessive sweating, feelings of weakness, dizziness or faintness, headache, hunger, abdominal pain, irritability and mood swings, palpitations, trembling, impaired vision. There may be sudden drowsiness or sudden awakening from sleep, especially accompanied by other symptoms.

In a person with diabetes, an insulin reaction should be treated by administering a rapidly absorbed source of sugar. Diabetics can learn how to recognise and handle hypoglycaemia.

Among non-diabetics, clinical hypoglycaemia is rare because the hormonal feedback systems that control the body's release of insulin are very efficient. When the body senses that blood glucose is low, the pancreas reacts by halting insulin secretion and other systems, aimed at maintaining an adequate supply of glucose, come into play. Diet can 'trick' the body into producing too much insulin and consequently experiencing some of the symptoms associated with hypoglycaemia. This occurs most often among women who consume a low-calorie, high-carbohydrate diet.

Typically a woman will have a carbohydrate breakfast – for example, orange juice, sugared tea or coffee and bread and jam. The pancreas will secrete a large amount of insulin to handle the large amount of glucose produced by this meal. But since the breakfast contained very little protein and fat, which take longer to metabolise than simple carbohydrates, by lunchtime the glucose from breakfast has been burned up and the woman may well experience some of the symptoms of hypoglycaemia: headache, hunger, shakiness, lightheadedness, irritability and palpitations, If she eases her hunger with a sweet snack or more simple carbohydrate, the pancreas will again respond by pumping out insulin; by late afternoon, the blood glucose may again be below normal and the symptoms will return.

This woman's body is reacting normally to poor diet. Although her blood sugar falls significantly, this type of reactive hypoglycaemia is normal variation rather than clinical, but she needs to attend to her diet. The symptoms can be avoided by adding protein and fat to her breakfast or by eating a snack mid-morning to take care of the large amount of insulin produced by the high-sugar breakfast. With such a simple solution it is pointless going from doctor to doctor to find a diagnosis for these symptoms.

Other causes of hypoglycaemia

Hypoglycaemia occurs in some diseases but, in contrast to reactive hypoglycaemia, the symptoms do not occur in response to eating carbohydrates. Instead, they may appear at unpredictable times, even when fasting. The most common cause of hypoglycaemia is sulfonylureas (oral anti-diabetes drugs) which increase insulin secretion and lower blood glucose.

Alcohol can create hypoglycaemia by interfering with the liver's ability to make glucose, particularly among people who drink heavily for several hours without eating. Other drugs that can lower blood glucose include large amounts of aspirin, acetaminophen, colchicine (a drug used to treat gout), MAO inhibitors, beta blockers, and some of the anti-psychotic medications.

Insulin-secreting tumours can also produce it through their abnormal hormone production. Most are insulinomas, small, usually benign, growths of pancreatic islet cells. Some cancers cause it, particularly of the liver and adrenal glands, carcinoid tumours, lymphoma, sarcoma and other relatively rare diseases. Liver and kidney diseases, severe infection and congestive heart failure also may produce hypoglycaemia.

Sometimes the excessive insulin is due to a faulty regulatory mechanism. Instead of the body sensing that it has enough insulin, the signals get mixed up and the pancreas continues to secrete the hormone. Hormonal imbalances, such as deficiencies of growth hormone or cortisone, also may cause it.

Prolonged fasting, especially in infants, can be a cause and newborn babies are particularly susceptible, especially in the first few hours of life before their glucose regulatory systems are fully operational. Babies born to women with poorly controlled diabetes may also have problems regulating blood sugar because their foetal pancreases have been producing large amounts of insulin to compensate for the high level of glucose in the mother's circulation. Infant hypoglycaemia may also be caused by congenital deficiencies in enzymes needed to metabolise glucose.

It should be stressed that hypoglycaemia from these miscellaneous causes should not be confused with the hypoglycaemia that is unrelated to food absorption and is potentially life-threatening. Its cause should be identified and treated as soon as possible. Fortunately, these are uncommon disorders.

Summing up

Diabetes is the most common of all endocrine disorders. It is also one of the most serious. Increased understanding of how to match insulin to diet and lifestyle, along with simple self-monitoring tests, have improved diabetes control. Most experts believe that better long-term control of diabetes will help to prevent many of the common complications of the disease. Hypoglycaemia that is unrelated to the treatment of diabetes is not as common as many people have been led to believe. Most cases are caused by poor diet.

CHAPTER ELEVEN

Thyroid Disorders

The thyroid, a butterfly-shaped gland that rests atop the windpipe, is the body's equivalent to a car's accelerator. Its hormones control the body's metabolic rate – when levels are too high body processes are speeded up, making you feel you are constantly running in high gear or, when hormone levels are too low, as though you are in low gear.

The thyroid normally weighs about 20g (0.7oz) but when diseased it may grow to many times that size. Thyroid overgrowth, goitre, is still very common and more frequent – at one in 10 – for women as compared to men. The thyroid enlarges in pregnancy and women who live in a region where goitre is common have a much higher incidence of goitres in pregnancy.

The thyroid hormones

There are two active thyroid hormones: triiodothyronine (T3), and thyroxine (T4). The numbers refer to the number of iodine atoms on each molecule, but how they differ in function is not known. T3 is the more active and a large portion of T4 is converted into T3. The hormones are stored in the thyroid until needed by the body, and when they fall too low the pituitary secretes thyroid-stimulating hormone (TSH) to tell the thyroid to increase hormone secretion and production (see Figure 18).

The thyroid hormones affect most metabolic processes and consumption of energy (calories), stimulate growth, lower cholesterol,

172

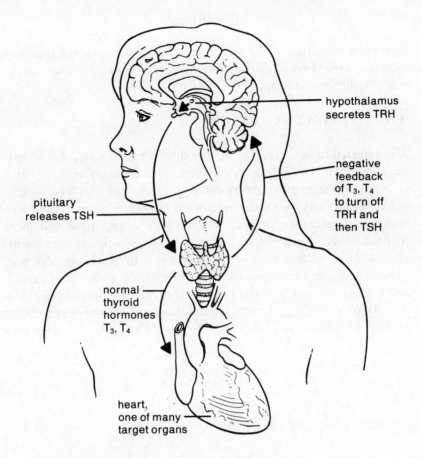

Figure 18. *The normal thyroid, its controls and activities*

develop the central nervous system, enhance the action of adrenal stress hormones and speed up the action of insulin.

There are several types of thyroid disease and virtually all of them are more common among women than men. Hyperthyroidism means a condition in which there are high levels of hormones; hypothyroidism is the opposite, but both can cause a goitre. A goitre can also be caused by a faulty pituitary gland telling a normal thyroid to over-produce and grow bigger.

Iodine deficiency has been a major cause of thyroid disease but this has been countered by iodine added to salt and greater consumption of seafoods. But excess iodine and undue stress may cause thyroid disease. Female sex hormones are thought to promote thyroid disorders and so pregnancy may mask them. Certain antibodies in the immune system may have an effect similar to TSH, making the thyroid overproduce. Exposure to X-rays or other ionising radiation can reduce the thyroid's ability to produce hormones and increase the risk of later thyroid cancer.

The hyperactive thyroid

Also referred to as Graves' disease or diffuse toxic goitre, this is characterised by a speeded-up metabolism with different effects. There seems to be a strong hereditary connection and sufferers have a rapid pulse, weight loss, muscular weakness, fatigue, irritability and nervousness, intolerance to heat, excessive sweating, loose and more frequent stools, hunger and shakiness. Hair growth and loss speeds up, and bald patches may occur, with the skin becoming very soft, thinner and more transparent, while fingernails grow more rapidly and have grooves. The eyeballs also appear to be enlarged but this is because of a swelling of tissue behind them and they appear to bulge because the upper eyelids become elevated. The protruding eyes may

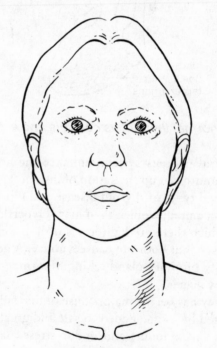

Figure 19. Development of a goitre: characteristic neck swelling and protruding eyes in Graves' disease

174

become inflamed and the bulging can damage the optic nerve and interfere with vision. Women may develop menstrual abnormalities, with longer or shorter gaps between periods; ovulation may stop, though there may be periodic menstrual bleeding, and there may be fertility problems.

The cause of Graves' disease is thyroid-stimulating antibodies and a tumour may develop in the shape of a horseshoe on the throat, just where the thyroid is.

There is a range of blood tests now which can check out levels in the thyroid and the pituitary to localise the cause of over- or under-production of hormone in either, because of their relationship mentioned earlier.

A young person with mild symptoms may be given extra thyroid hormone to see if this will lower TSH production and so lower the thyroid's hormone input. There is a newer test which looks at the way the hypothalamus controls pituitary and thyroid and so show any difference between them.

Other types of hyperthyroidism

About 30 per cent of hyperthyroidism is due to one or more 'hot' nodules in which specific areas of the gland become overactive. Five per cent of cases will have one nodule and 25 per cent multiple nodules, which usually show up in a thyroid scan. The rest of the gland gradually stops functioning and so one part may feel enlarged; where there are several nodules the gland will feel enlarged and lumpy.

A patient may develop flu-like symptoms with a sore throat due to an inflamed thyroid, making it tender, and excessive hormones are secreted into the blood. Blood tests will show high levels of thyroid hormone. While the gland may feel enlarged, there will be a low uptake of radioactive iodine and scans will be normal. This inflammatory form usually subsides after a few weeks. Part of that recovery may lead to lower production of hormone (hypothyroidism) but this also returns to normal.

In rare cases tumours can cause hyperthyroidism with excessive TSH causing hyperactivity. The tumours can include those of the reproductive system. The treatment is to remove the source of the abnormal hormone production.

If a person has thyroid nodules, then consuming too much iodine in the diet can lead to hyperthyroidism but there really has to be a large intake over a lengthy period of time. If you start consuming enormous amounts of seaweed, or kelp, or thyroid pills as part of a diet to lose weight then you can expect problems. Moderation and treatment under someone who knows your needs is important.

Treatment of hyperthyroidism

Anti-thyroid drugs, radioactive iodine and surgery are all means of treating hyperthyroidism. The drugs prevent the gland from manu-facturing hormone and are preferred for children; they are carbimazole or propylthiouracil (PTU). They may be given for up to a year or more.

Radioactive iodine is used to destroy part of the thyroid – the patient taking a drink containing radioactive iodine, the iodine taking it directly to the thyroid. The isotopes decay in a few days or are cleared through the urine. The isotopes destroy part of the thyroid to prevent any cancer cell growth. Because iodine is so specific it will only take the radioactive isotopes to the thyroid so no risk has been found of them damaging other parts of the body. But this treatment should not be given to a pregnant or breastfeeding mother because it will work through to the foetus or baby. Thyroid replacement hormones may be needed after treatment to make up for any loss, or, of course, where it was necessary to destroy all of the thyroid.

Surgically, enough of the thyroid is removed so that it produces normal, not raised, levels of hormone. But it is normally only done on patients who are otherwise well. Surgeons also have to make sure that they do not damage the parathyroid glands, or affect the nearby nerves which are important for speech. If the parathyroids are damaged, replacement hormone will be needed to metabolise calcium.

Beta-blocking drugs, such as propanalol, may be given during treatment to help control symptoms such as palpitations and ner-vousness. The eye problems accompanying Graves' disease may be treated with steroids to reduce the swelling behind the eyeball and lessen the bulging, and to counter eye inflammation. Frequently, patients who experience a remission of Graves' disease with anti-thyroid drugs will eventually develop hypothyroidism, and require replacement hormones.

The underactive thyroid

Hypothyroidism, a deficiency of thyroid hormone may take years to develop, producing increasingly troublesome symptoms. Yet, once diagnosed, it is easily treated with replacement hormone.

It is most serious in infants and very young children. Babies and children may have stunted growth and delayed sexual development. A test for thyroid hormone at birth can be done on the umbilical cord.

In hypothyroidism, body processes slow down, causing fatigue and listlessness. The first sign may be development of a goitre caused by the pituitary producing large amounts of TSH in an effort to stimulate the thyroid into action.

Women notice that their skin becomes coarser, very dry and scaly, particularly over the elbows and on the legs. It will feel cold and clammy to the touch and there is a lack of sweating. Nails are slow-growing, dry and brittle. The hair thins and becomes coarser. Constipation, premature greying (before the age of 30) and vitiligo – patches of white, unpigmented skin – are common.

While complaining of loss of appetite, women may still gain weight despite eating less. The eyelids and face often become puffy. A woman's voice may become deeper and husky, symptoms often mistaken for laryngitis. Heavy menstrual periods and infertility, both caused by a lack of ovulation are common, and both men and women may experience a loss of interest in sex and most other activities.

Impaired hearing or loss of balance may occur, and while a slow heart rate is more common, there may be palpitations. Stiffness in the joints, especially in the morning is also common and may be mistaken for arthritis or rheumatism. As it progresses, full-blown myxoedema may develop with a thickening of facial features, overgrowth of the tongue, generalised swelling or oedema, extreme lethargy, mental dullness and impaired memory. Untreated it may progress to myxoedema coma and even death.

At one time iodine deficiency was the commonest cause of hypothyroidism but over-consumption through fad diets can also cause it. Also a pregnant woman taking too much iodine can cause the condition and goitre in the baby. Lithium (a drug used to treat manic depression) can also produce it, as can iodine-dye X-rays in hypersensitive people.

Also common is Hashimoto's disease in older children and adults, with chronic inflammation of the thyroid without infection and enlargement of the gland. Many women begin to notice they are developing a goitre when a favourite necklace suddenly feels too tight. This condition appears to be inherited, but is more common amongst women; the body produces antibodies against its thyroid tissue and it is different from other forms of hypothyroidism because of this.

Treatment of hypothyroidism

This is usually with thyroxine pills. Originally made from animal extract, their composition was not constant, so their activity was variable. They caused surges which could have led to palpitations and so be dangerous for those with an underlying heart disease.

Thyroid cancer

This is relatively rare and responds very well to treatment – in a sense it is one of the best cancers to have. In some countries there seems to be an increase in its incidence. This may perhaps be due to the large number of children and adolescents between the 1920s and 1960s who were given X-rays for a range of minor ailments before adequate research on radiation dosages was put into practice. People exposed to radiation from atomic bomb tests or other nuclear incidents also have a higher rate of thyroid cancer; but again, cure rates, after treatment, are very good. There is a need for preventive research in this area by radiographers so that certain groups can check out whether they do in fact run a higher risk from the early overdoses of X-rays.

Summing up

Thyroid disease, whether causing too much or too little thyroid hormone, affects virtually every system and process in the body. It may go undiagnosed for long periods because the symptoms are often vague or easily mistaken for other conditions. Since many of these disorders tend to be hereditary, anyone with a family history of thyroid disease should be particularly attuned to early warning signs. Thyroid disease, whether of under- or over-activity, is simple to treat. Thyroid cancer can also be treated easily and cured, so this is a good example of why cancer should not inspire fear.

CHAPTER TWELVE

Disorders of the Adrenal Glands

The adrenals are a pair of triangular glands that rest on top of the kidneys. The outer yellowish portion, the adrenal cortex, manufactures cortisone and other steroid hormones. The inner, reddish brown portion is called the adrenal medulla, and it secretes catecholamines, noradrenaline and adrenaline (norepinephrine and epinephrine), the so-called stress hormones. Both the adrenal cortex and medulla functions are regulated by intricate feedback systems that control numerous body functions.

The steroid hormones

Three different groups of steroid hormones are secreted by the adrenal cortex: the corticosteroids, which include hydrocortisone, the mineralocorticoids (primarily aldosterone) and the sex steroids, namely androgen, oestrogen and progesterone. (The sex hormones are produced in larger quantities by the male testes and the female ovaries.)

All of the steroid hormones are synthesised from cholesterol. A certain amount of cholesterol is essential to all animal life. Too much produced or taken in means the body may not be able to handle the excess; it builds up in the blood and forms the fatty deposits that lead to hardening of the arteries and clogging of the coronary blood vessels.

Proper function of the adrenal cortex depends upon extremely sensitive hormonal feedback interactions with other glands. The secretion of the adrenals' glucocorticoids and sex steroids, for example, is controlled by the pituitary's production of ACTH, while the production of aldosterone, to control salt and water balance, is regulated by the renin-angiotensin system.

Corticosteroid secretion is closely linked to our individual bio-rhythms or internal clocks. Steroid secretion is lowest during the four hours before going to bed and the first two hours of sleep; it then rises to peak at about wake-up time. Blood levels of corticosteroids are highest in the early morning, gradually falling during the day, with periodic pulses that coincide with our feelings of renewed energy. This internal biological clock is closely tied to light/dark, sleep/wake and feeding cycles. We are perhaps most acutely aware of our bio-logical clocks, or diurnal rhythm, when we fly across several time zones. Jet lag is a function of our diurnal rhythm, and it usually takes several days to reset our internal biological clock to coincide with the new time zone. There is now evidence that jet lag is linked to the dis-turbed activity of the pineal gland. Research studies are giving participants one of the substances produced by the thyroid.

Many factors can alter secretion of adrenal steroids including illness, psychological stress, infection, fever, exposure to cold or heat, increased physical activity and certain drugs. Whenever the body is subjected to any kind of stress, the adrenal glands respond by increas-ing output of corticosteroids as well as stress hormones. If not, blood pressure can fall dangerously and cardiovascular collapse or shock may result, leading to death. So, a person on long-term steroid therapy, such as prednisolone treatment of chronic asthma, cannot abruptly stop taking the drugs.

Topical steroids that are applied to the skin may be absorbed in sufficient amounts to affect normal adrenal function. Just because they can be bought over the counter in certain formulations does not mean to say that they should be treated lightly, and they should be used spar-ingly, preferably under medical supervision, although women are particularly good at spotting any adverse reactions before their doctors. Whenever steroid medications are given over a period of time, the pituitary gland becomes accustomed to the high levels of steroids and stops producing ACTH (whose function is to tell the adrenals to secrete their coricosteroids). If the drugs are then stopped and the person is exposed to a normal stress, they may go into shock because the adrenals are still 'asleep'. This complication of steroid therapy can be avoided, in some conditions, by using a short-acting drug, such as prednisolone, and administering it at eight every other morning instead of every day. This regime follows the body's normal early morning peak pulse of hydrocortisone secretion, and the alternate administration is not as likely to suppress the normal feedback system.

Birth control pills which are high in oestrogen raise steroid levels, which also can lead to swelling and increased blood pressure from the excess sodium and fluid. These side effects were more common with the earlier pills, which contained more oestrogen. The hormonal changes of pregnancy are similar to those of the pill. Some women's adrenal glands produce very high levels of corticosteroids, which can lead to symptoms similar to those seen in patients with Cushing's syndrome – reddish stretch marks, a rounding of the face, fluid retention and mild glucose intolerance. Over-production of adrenal hormones may also be related to toxaemia in pregnancy, but this has not been proved.

Several congenital errors can cause over- or under-production of adrenal hormones. Enzyme deficiency can cause overgrowth of the adrenal cortex and excessive production of androgen. This causes virilisation of females and false, precocious puberty in males. It is called either the adreno-genital syndrome or congenital adrenal hyperplasia. It is a surprisingly common condition. Since this condition can be treated, women who would not otherwise have conceived will be fertile if given the appropriate therapy. Another inborn metabolic error causes inadequate aldosterone, and so excessive loss of salt and water and low blood pressure. Defects in glucocorticoid production, especially hydrocortisone, interfere with the metabolism of food and numerous other body functions.

Secretion of corticosteroids is closely related to production of growth hormone. Growth hormone is suppressed in people with chronically high levels of steroids, which is believed to explain the stunted growth in children who are treated with long-term steroids for asthma, juvenile arthritis and other chronic disorders. Or the body may see the cortisone as similar enough to a sex steroid hormone that it is 'tricked' into thinking that the child has become an adult and therefore should stop growing. The steroid closes the growth plates of the long bones.

Cushing's syndrome

One of the most common disorders of the adrenal cortex, occurring more often in women than men, Cushing's syndrome can appear at any age, but most often between 20 and 40, frequently during or immediately after pregnancy.

Excessive hairiness, unexplained weight gain and changes in the distribution of body fat are the symptoms usually associated with Cushing's. The face becomes moon-shaped and body fat accumulates on the trunk, especially on the abdomen and upper back causing 'buffalo hump'. The skin also becomes very thin, bruising easily and disfigured by purplish stretch marks. Muscle weakness, menstrual irregularity and infertility are also common.

Tests usually show abnormal glucose metabolism, and many people develop diabetes. The body's chemical balance is upset. Excessive sodium retention causes swelling and hypertension, while a loss of potassium accounts for the muscle weakness. Cuts and other wounds are very slow in healing and abnormal calcium metabolism leads to thinning and weakening of the bones, explaining why stress fractures are common among Cushing's patients.

A common, induced cause of Cushing's, is overuse of steroid medicines to treat asthma, arthritis and other chronic diseases. Steroid creams for external use can also produce it and, in such cases, treatment involves a gradual weaning away from the steroids.

A hormone-producing tumour or overgrowth of the adrenal gland may cause too much hydrocortisone. Treatment entails surgical removal of the source of the abnormal hormone production, such as a diseased adrenal gland, followed by hormone treatments to restore the pituitary's normal production of ACTH. This will eventually 'wake up' the remaining adrenal gland and stimulate it to produce hydrocortisone.

The problem may be located in the pituitary and hypothalamus, resulting in an overproduction of ACTH. This stimulates the adrenals to secrete too much hydrocortisone and is treated by correcting the pituitary-hypothalamic disorder.

When hormone levels are normal again, electrolysis may be needed to remove the hairiness that has already occurred. Further thinning of the bones may be prevented, but established osteoporosis is difficult or impossible to reverse.

Addison's disease

Addisons's disease, the opposite of Cushing's syndrome, is caused by a chronic deficiency of adrenal hormones. In more than half of such cases, the adrenal cortex has wasted away. Most commonly, this is caused by an auto-immune disorder in which, for unknown reasons, the body produces antibodies against one or more organs, resulting in their destruction. The second most common cause is infection, usually tuberculosis, which causes death and calcification of the adrenal tissue. Most of these patients have never been diagnosed as having tuberculosis, but careful medical investigation will often turn up signs of an inactive infection, usually in the lungs.

Other causes of adrenal failure include fungal infections – such as histoplasmosis, coccidioidomycosis, blastomycosis – meningitis, and failure of the pituitary. Symptoms become evident when about 95 per cent of the adrenal gland has been destroyed. These include increasing weakness, fatigue, severe muscle cramps, weight loss, darkening of the skin, low blood pressure, loss of appetite, low blood sugar, abdominal pain, nausea and vomiting. It is the fatigue and lightheadedness which normally takes people to the doctor. The skin's signs are useful: a summer tan may not fade, the pigmented mucosal lining in a woman's genital area takes on a blue-grey colour and there may be dark creases on the palms, and more freckles and moles on the upper body. It may also be highlighted by patches of unpigmented white skin (vitiligo) where it is exposed to the sun.

Addison's disease also affects sexual function with desire decreasing and some men experiencing impotence. In women there may be thinning of the pubic and under-arm hair due to decreased androgens, and menstrual irregularity and infertility are also common.

But, treatment with daily hormone replacement enables sufferers to live a normal life. Hydrocortisone in replacement doses has few side effects. A mineralocorticoid (such as fludrocortisone) may be needed to balance blood pressure and fluid balance.

Conn's syndrome

This is very rare compared to the other conditions mentioned. It is caused by an overproduction of aldosterone due to a benign tumour of the gland with mild, higher blood pressure, excessive urination and potassium depletion. For the doctor the issue is deciding whether the problem arises from an adrenal tumour or a kidney disorder. Treatment may require surgical removal of the tumour.

Virilising syndromes

The adrenal glands produce small amounts of androgen which the body turns into testosterone in both male and female. A small excess of this can cause virilisation, in which girls develop male characteristics and boys experience premature sexual development. This is a rare condition and is caused by an insufficiency, or defect, in one of the enzymes needed to synthesise hyrodrocortisone. Treatment is with steroids, such as prednisolone, to suppress the excessive adrenal activity.

Disorders of the adrenal medulla

The major hormones secreted by the adrenal medulla – noradrenaline (norepinephrine) and adrenaline (epinephrine) – are responsible for our fight-or-flight response. When the body sees danger, including internal stress, the adrenal medulla starts producing them. They give the surge to help us escape or cope with the threat. The heart speeds up, the smallest arteries constrict to raise blood pressure and the muscles get extra blood. Oxygen uptake is increased and the liver and muscles convert stored glycogen for immediate energy, while insulin is shut off to keep the blood glucose level right up for energy.

The over-competitive, 'type A' person seems to secrete large amounts of the hormones in response to even very minor stresses, which is why some argue they may have more heart attacks. They may be damaging the vessels and causing a buildup of fatty deposits along the artery walls.

Although catecholamines are usually associated with stress roles, they have many other functions. They regulate body fluid, electrolyte balance, cell growth and division, regulation of the nervous system and muscle function, secretion of various proteins and fat metabolism. They generate body heat by promoting shivering and mobilise stored fuel for the muscles during exercise.

Orthostatic hypotension

When we get up from a sitting or lying position our circulatory system constricts to prevent falling blood pressure, so ensuring a continuity of supply to the brain. The nervous system makes the blood vessels react in this way. This is linked to the work of the catecholamines. If this feedback system is not in tune, then we may experience a temporary drop in blood pressure when getting up and this is called orthostatic hypotension. Drugs used to treat high blood pressure may also cause this, as may certain nerve disorders.

Commonsense can sort this out – less haste, less dizziness by moving smoothly, sleeping with your head up, etc. But if it is drug-induced, then you need to consult your doctor about an alternative. Where it is more disabling, people may wear elasticated stockings to prevent a pooling of the blood in the legs. A mineralocorticoid drug, such as fludrocortisone, along with a high intake of salt to expand blood volume may also be recommended.

Phaeochromocytoma

This is a tumour, usually benign, which produces catecholamines, resulting in high blood pressure. They are rare, accounting for only one per cent of all cases of hypertension, and easily removed to effect a cure. Because it can cause high hypertension it can do severe damage to eyes and kidneys and it usually does not respond to conventional drugs. There may also be angina and severe heart attack but without evidence of coronary disease. Others symptoms include: severe headaches, excessive sweating, palpitations, nausea and vomiting, tremor, weakness, fatigue, nervousness and anxiety, indigestion, hot flushes, numbness or tingling, blurred vision, dizziness, fainting and a variety of pains. Sometimes this stress is associated with mild diabetes because catecholamines act against insulin.

Codeine (and other opiate-based drugs) and some other painkillers and anaesthetics can produce a fatal reaction to excess catecholamines. Severe reactions may be produced by histamines, ACTH and glucagon, as may substances used in some X-ray procedures. A severe rise in blood pressure may occur with certain anti-cold formulations and decongestants and drugs such as guanethidine and tricyclic antidepressants. These should be avoided if phaeochromocytoma is suspected. It can also accompany other disorders such as rare thyroid tumours as well as neurofibromas. More commonly however, the tumour develops directly in the adrenal medulla itself alone. The majority, some 95 per cent, are benign, and the remaining malignant five per cent have metastases to the bone and liver.

Diagnosis is by X-ray or the new CAT scans which have displaced X-rays, or challenging the possible tumour with glucagon or similar to stimulate catecholamine release and see if there is a rise in blood pressure. After surgical removal most patients recover fully and again have normal blood pressure.

Summing up

The adrenal glands produce a number of hormones that affect virtually every system and function in the body. Their release is controlled by intricate feedback systems but may also be influenced by stress, both internal and external. Once a diagnosis has been done, though it may be lengthy, most adrenal disorders can be successfully treated.

CHAPTER THIRTEEN

Eating Disorders

Either too much or too little weight is one of our most common health problems. This can profoundly affect a woman's endocrine system, causing menstrual irregularities, infertility and other hormonal problems.

Obesity

To determine whether a person is obese, you can carry out a skin-fold test. She/he can be weighed under water to determine percentage of body fat versus bones. There are also complicated formulae to calculate body mass index, uptake of inert gases, total bodywater or potassium. For most, this is unnecessary: use the mirror or the bathroom scales to see if you look or are overweight. You can also check against a height-to-weight scale for your age group.

Nutritionists are still debating whether obesity is genetically or environmentally determined. Many overweight people say they are so because of their 'fat' genes – based on seeing thin people eat enormous amounts without their getting fat. But then even if a person has inherited a tendency to be fat, the excess will still generally come from taking in more calories than they burn up. Unless there is a serious underlying problem correct weight can be maintained by a balance of diet and exercise. Parents should start this off with their children at a young age – overweight children tend to grow into overweight adults and have life-long problems. Sedentary lifestyles lead to overweight, even though the person may eat less than an active colleague. Eating habits may be a factor; an overweight person eats

Table 6 : Weight guide for women

Height without shoes		Ideal weight range (without clothes)	
cm	ft in	kg	lb
147	4 10	42–51	92–112
150	4 11	43–53	95–116
152	5 0	44–54	97–119
155	5 1	45–55	100–122
157	5 2	47–57	103–126
160	5 3	48–59	106–130
162	5 4	50–62	110–135
165	5 5	51–63	114–139
167	5 6	53–65	117–144
170	5 7	56–67	121–148
172	5 8	57–69	125–152
175	5 9	58–71	128–157
177	5 10	60–73	132–161
180	5 11	62–74	136–165
182	6 0	63–75	139–170

rapidly, while the thin person eats slowly, allowing the brain's hunger centre time to react to food intake and signal that it has been satisfied.

How many calories do you need?

A calorie is simply the amount of energy required to raise the temperature of one gram of water one degree centigrade. Your basal metabolic rate is the number of calories you need each day. The average woman weighing 60kg (135lb) needs somewhere between 1,300 and 1,600 calories a day to support her basic metabolic needs.

To calculate approximately how many calories a person may need to support basal metabolism and physical activities use the following:

Table 7:

Activity level	Calories per kg (lb)	
Very sedentary	24	(12)
Moderate	30	(15)
Vigorous	4	(20)

But everyone is different and metabolism gradually slows down with age, so we need less calories. There are a number of ways of calculating an individual's personal needs and you can get hold of a chart from your doctor, or local weight-watchers' group.

In determining whether a person is obese the amount of body fat must be taken into consideration. When we eat more than we burn up, the excess is stored as fat. There are two types of obesity: hyperplastic, in which the number of fat cells increases, and hypertrophic, in which the fat cells themselves become enlarged. Animal studies have found that, for some species, patterns of infant feeding determine the number of fat cells and presumably lead to hyperplastic obesity. For example, over-fed baby rats develop a greater number of fat cells than those fed a normal diet, but this has not been proved in humans.

Table 8: Calories Expended in Physical Activity

Activity	*Calories used per hour*
Strolling at 1mph	150
Walking at 2mph	200
Walking at 4mph	350
Jogging	600
Running	800–1000
Ballet exercises/calisthenics	300
Cycling at 5mph	250
Cycling at 10mph	450
Tennis (doubles)	350–450
Tennis (singles)	400–500
Swimming (breast or backstroke)	300–600
Swimming (crawl)	700–900
Aerobic dancing	600–800
Cross-country skiing	700–1000

Overweight babies have larger than normal fat cells, but it is not known when this increase takes place. A fat cell forms for life, although it will shrink with weight loss. However, the 'starved' fat cell may send forth hunger signals, which would explain why most people resume over-eating after losing weight.

A person who is very muscular and large-boned may weigh much more than recommended on a standard table, and still not be obese.

A rugby player's weight may be more than 20 per cent above that on a weight table, and still be below average in total body fat. On average, fat makes up 5 to 10 per cent of the weight of a lean man, and 10 to 20 per cent of the weight of a lean woman. Obese for a woman means 30 per cent overweight.

Health risks of obesity

Generally overweight people die earlier than their ideal-weight counterparts, with increased risk of heart attacks, strokes, high blood pressure, diabetes, respiratory disorders, gallstones and cancers, especially those of the breast and uterus. They are more accident-prone, perhaps because they tend to be awkward and have slower reactions.

An overweight person may have low self-esteem and, not uncommonly, emotional problems. Rather than being jolly, obese people are more likely to be unhappy and to perceive themselves as being weak-willed and unattractive. Fashions are designed for a svelte figure. A thin person is more likely to get a job and a promotion than an equally-qualified fat person. Surveys have even found that thin people tend to be paid more than those who are overweight!

Women, all too often, turn to crash or fad diets to lose unwanted weight. Many lose weight, but up to 95 per cent quickly regain what they lost while dieting. This sudden weight gain not only makes the fat cells fat again, but actually causes them to multiply.

Most weight-loss schemes are based on a calorie-restricted eating plan that is difficult to maintain for very long and does not address faulty eating problems that have been built over a lifetime. The body's protective mechanisms quickly react by increasing hunger signals and re-setting the basal metabolic rate to conserve energy. Hunger ensures that the body has a steady supply of energy to carry out its vital functions; hunger is almost impossible to ignore if food is available.

The body also tries to protect itself from starvation. It does not recognise the difference between a diet and involuntary starvation in a concentration camp or that caused by famine. So it will reduce its metabolic rate to conserve energy and start to break down lean body tissue, mostly muscles, and convert this into blood glucose. This is another good reason why fasting and extreme low-calorie diets should be avoided unless carried out under very close medical supervision.

Tedious as it may sound, the safest and most effective way to lose excessive weight is a moderate reduction in calories and an increase in exercise. This may be more difficult than going on a crash diet, but it works. Remember that walking is still one of the best of all exercises.

You should not try to lose more than 1.5kg (2–3lb) a week. In order to lose 450g (1lb) you must burn up 3,500 more calories than consumed. So by eating 700 fewer calories a day and increasing exercise enough to burn up an additional 300 calories, a person can lose almost 1kg (2lb) a week. A dieter needs at least 1,000 calories a day, including foods from the four basic food groups to ensure adequate nutrition. Simply cutting portion size, reducing the amount of fat in the diet (one gram of fat contains nine calories compared to four calories per gram in carbohydrates and protein), and increasing the amount of complex carbohydrates and fibre (which has a filling effect and helps prevent feeling hungry), is usually sufficient for most people who want to lose a moderate amount of weight. Check with your doctor or local health education promotion unit for various leaflets on sensible nutrition and dieting.

Hormone-related causes of obesity

Steroid hormones promote weight gain and a redistribution of fat deposits. People with Cushing's syndrome and those on long-term steroid drugs will develop a rounded, moon-shaped face, a layer of fat on the upper back (often called buffalo hump), weight gain on the trunk and upper body, accompanied by a thinning of the arms and legs. They feel ravenously hungry; the hormones promote fluid retention, which adds to bloating and weight gain.

Thyroid deficiency may cause moderate weight gain from fluid retention. The slowed-down metabolism also means less calories are burned up, resulting in their being stored as body fat. An overactive thyroid may cause loss of weight, even though food consumption may be increased. Some women can actually gain weight because they are hungry all the time and eat more calories than their body can burn up.

Marked obesity in children may be caused by a variety of genetic disorders affecting the endocrine system. Mental retardation and other defects accompany many of these syndromes, which tend to be quite rare. Brain tumours or infections affecting the hypothalamus and pituitary also can cause childhood obesity, but these are usually accompanied by other telltale symptoms.

Obesity and the endocrine system

Hormonal balance is affected by obesity and can result in serious endocrine diseases. Type 2, insulin-resistant diabetes, is one of the most common of these. The excessive fatty tissue seems to cause increased insulin resistance and Type 2 diabetics produce an excessive amount of insulin, but the hormone is not utilised.

Overweight women frequently experience extra hair growth, menstrual irregularity and infertility due to increased conversion of androgen to oestrogen in fatty tissue. After menopause, the excessive androgens, and their conversion to oestrogens, are believed to account for the increased risk of uterine cancer found among obese women.

Obesity lowers production of growth hormone, but does not appear to alter production of other pituitary hormones. Among men, obesity lowers testosterone levels and increases oestrogens. These changes usually are not apparent, though there are instances in which they prompt the growth of breast tissue, impotence and feminisation.

Weight-loss techniques

Correcting the underlying endocrine disease will usually resolve the weight problem, although dieting may be necessary to lose the accumulated fat. But secondary obesity is uncommon. Most overweight is due to overeating and under-exercising.

Use of diuretics, appetite suppressants or laxatives is not a good idea for a healthy person trying to lose weight. Surgery, in which varying amounts of the stomach or intestines are removed, or the temporary stapling off of a portion of the intestinal tract, is intended for people whose massive overweight is virtually life-threatening.

A procedure in which a balloon is inserted into the stomach and then partially inflated to give a feeling of fullness can cause problems if it suddenly deflates. This strategy should be accompanied by a programme to change eating behaviour so the weight is not regained when the balloon is deflated and removed.

Surgical removal of layers of fat is sometimes done, but these are complicated operations that may cause permanent damage to nerves and blood vessels. The so-called 'tummy tuck,' in which some plastic surgeons remove some abdominal fat and tighten tummy muscles, is increasingly popular. But this should not be considered a treatment for obesity. It is really a cosmetic procedure to remove a sagging fold of skin, left after weight loss, particularly in older people.

Similarly, fat suction operations, in which a saline solution is injected into a layer of fat which is then vacuumed out, has become a common plastic surgery technique in the US and France (where it was developed). This procedure does not seem to have as many potentially serious complications as surgical removal of fat, but it works only on relatively small areas; it may be less effective in older individuals and is not recommended for people who are more than a few pounds overweight.

Increased physical activity is almost as important as reduced food intake. Sadly, many overweight women are embarrassed to join exercise classes because they feel ungainly and out-of-place. Simply recognising that you are not alone, losing weight and adopting a healthier, more active lifestyle in the company of others can be a major step forward towards life-long weight control.

Anorexia nervosa and bulimia

Only recently have two distressingly common eating disorders been brought to widespread public attention. Both anorexia nervosa and bulimia appear to be most evident in young women – they are generally of above average intelligence and the upper socio-economic strata. Their bizarre eating behaviour disrupts families and often leads to death through self-starvation.

Records of anorexic cases go back hundreds of years, so the condition is not new, but its cause remains unknown. Most agree this extreme, life-threatening disease includes serious emotional problems. Some researchers believe that the hypothalamus may be involved. A young woman may be schizophrenic or suffering from serious paranoia or obsessive behaviour, but this is not a common denominator.

Deep-seated family problems have been implicated in various eating disorders, such as anorexia, bulimia and obesity, where parents and children seem constantly to be involved in each other's problems. In a simpler sense, both anorexia and bulimia may be learned behaviour, usually during the teenage years. Anorexia is becoming more common, especially among upper-class young women in developed countries. For unexplained reasons, a disproportionate number are Jewish. Occasionally, a young man will develop anorexia, but less than six per cent of cases are men. However, young male athletes may take to compulsive exercising so they can eat huge amounts of food.

Anorexia and bulimia may occur independently or together. Since our society prizes thinness, and large numbers of young women seem eternally to be trying to lose weight, it is sometimes difficult to distinguish between obsessive dieting and true anorexia nervosa. Family and friends may notice that a young woman is losing weight, but often do not associate it with illness. She, herself, may be overly concerned with health and fitness. Many anorexics turn to excessive, compulsive exercise to increase weight loss, a move that may be interpreted as healthy.

Typically, the first visit to the doctor is for failure to menstruate, caused by the hormonal changes accompanying weight loss. The classic symptoms used by physicians to diagnose anorexia nervosa include:

1 A loss of a quarter or more of body weight. No physical illness can be found to explain the weight loss.
2 A distorted body image and obsessive fear of being fat. The young woman will insist that she feels or looks fat, even though she may be emaciated.
3 Distorted preoccupation with food and eating. Anorexics will often spend hours preparing elaborate meals or obsessively collect recipes. They will then not eat what they have prepared, taking a morsel or two and then insisting they are full.
4 Signs of starvation. Doctors frequently use terms referring to a concentration camp or a famine to describe the physical appearance of an anorexic patient. This extreme thinness is not apparent when women are clothed because many, paradoxically, tend to dress to make themselves look fatter – choosing long-sleeved, fuller, styles – that disguise their emaciated bodies.

Other common symptoms, all associated with extreme malnutrition, include a low body temperature (hypothermia), low heart rate (bradycardia) and low blood pressure (hypotension). Extreme sensitivity to cold is common; when exposed to low temperatures, the women will feel numbness or tingling in their hand and feet. This is caused by constriction of the peripheral blood vessels as the body tries to conserve as much heat and energy as possible. Swelling from accumulation of fluid, another mark of starvation, also is common.

In investigating the family history of anorexic patients, doctors frequently find that the mothers, and occasionally the sisters as well, are markedly underweight. This is contrary to the popular notion that a young woman will starve herself because she has an obese mother, or other family members, and wants to avoid becoming fat herself. A study of over 100 anorexic patients found that only ten had family members who were overweight; in contrast, 29 had family members who were markedly underweight. In some cases, mothers who themselves have a history of anorexia impose strange eating patterns on their children.

Consequences of anorexia

It is important to recognise that this is a chronic disease with a high death rate. These unfortunate women have a distorted body image – they would rather die than gain weight. Many die of fatal arrhythmia, caused by the deterioration of the heart muscle. Breathing also becomes difficult because of weakened respiratory muscles.

Extreme malnutrition has numerous effects on the endocrine system, in addition to the most obvious, the cessation of menstruation. Everything slows down in an attempt to conserve energy. Production of the pituitary's gonad-stimulating hormones drops, as does production of the sex hormones. The thyroid lowers production of its hormones in an effort to slow metabolism.

Treatment involves hospitalisation, and often forced feeding. After the immediate danger of starvation is over, intensive psychiatric therapy can begin. It is a lengthy process, sometimes continuing for years. There is also a high relapse rate. Many women who have recovered still say they are uncomfortable about eating or their body image.

Follow-up studies have found that about half the anorexics achieve their normal weight within two years; some 20 per cent gain, but remain underweight; 6 per cent die and 5 per cent become obese. Menstruation recurs in between 50 to 75 per cent with the gain of weight, but irregularity of menstruation is common. Half the anorexic patients continue to have psychiatric or emotional problems serious enough to require treatment.

Bulimia

Bulimia, which means 'ox hunger,' is marked by a voracious, uncontrolled appetite. It often accompanies or follows anorexia. After periods of self-starvation, the woman becomes so hungry that she consumes quantities of food. Then the determination to stay thin takes over and purging is the next phase, usually by induced vomiting. With some bulimics, the vomiting becomes ritualistic.

Some bulimics attempt to compensate for a food binge by taking huge amounts of laxatives. Diuretic abuse is also common, and some, especially young people with poorly-controlled diabetes, may decrease their insulin dose to cause the sugar to pass into the urine. All of these are extremely risky, causing serious medical problems. Ironically, neither laxatives nor diuretics can control weight gain when massive amounts of food are consumed.

Unlike anorexia, bulimia is a new disorder. It seems particularly common among young women who are driven to succeed. Like anorexics, they are obsessed with a fear of getting fat, but they also have an irresistible urge to overeat. Some starve themselves, but will eventually binge, usually when they are alone, so that no-one can observe their compulsive eating. Some bulimics can consume up to 50,000 calories a day.

Bulimics seem to have a greater incidence of anti-social behaviour. One study found that 12 to 14 per cent of bulimics admitted to stealing, generally food. Drug and alcohol abuse, self-mutilation and suicide are also relatively common in this group.

Consequences of bulimia

Apart from the emotional and eating problems, bulimia does not have as many physical consequences as anorexia. The women are usually thin; some are overweight but the emaciation seen in anorexics is rare. The repeated vomiting and diarrhoea causes disturbances in body chemistry, particularly potassium depletion. This can cause convulsions, muscle spasms and weakness, but usually not to a serious extent.

Lack of menstruation sometimes occurs, but is not as common as in anorexia. Impaired taste and tooth decay are common. These are thought to be the result of the frequent exposure to gastric acids when vomiting. Sometimes the salivary glands enlarge.

Depression and emotional disorders are particularly common among bulimics. There are now many self-help groups that have been set up and many bulimic women with deep-seated emotional problems have found it useful to share their problems with people in similar situations.

Summing up

Obesity, anorexia and bulimia can all have serious consequences on emotional and physical health. Many believe that these disorders have their roots in childhood. Parents should instil sensible eating habits in their children and food should not be used for reproach or reward. Parents of teenage daughters should be particularly aware of weight loss, preoccupation with food and thinness and other warning signs, in their children.

CHAPTER FOURTEEN

How Hormones Affect Your Skin and Hair

The skin is a vital organ that provides the body with essential protective covering, serves as a sensory organ and performs a variety of metabolic and other functions. As mentioned at length earlier in this book, the skin can serve as an early warning area for various disorders, including those of the thyroid such as Addison's and Cushing's syndromes.

Hair is mostly dead tissue derived from the skin but it can be an important indicator of endocrine and other diseases.

Our preoccupation with beautifying skin and hair begins at an early age. It is important, however, that women select toiletries with correct information and a clear understanding of what they can do.

Skin anatomy and function

The skin is composed of two layers – the outer epidermis and the underlying dermis – both of which have several subdivisions. The epidermis gives rise to the nails and hair and also contains the sweat glands' pores, or openings.

Except on the palms of the hands and soles of the feet, the epidermis is paper thin and is made of five layers of different cells in most places. About 95 per cent of cells in the epidermis are keratinocytes, the body's protective outer layer which keep out harmful substances and prevent the loss of vital body fluids. The other 5 per cent of cells are melanocytes, pigment cells which give it its colour and protect the underlying tissue from the sun's ultraviolet rays.

The outermost layer of the epidermis is called the stratum corneum, a horny layer composed mostly of tough, opaque, keratin protein. The outer skin cells contain soft keratin and the protein which makes up the nails and hair is harder. All are actually dead cells that are constantly being worn off and replaced by cells moving up from the basal layer – the stratum germinativum. The basal layer is like a cell factory. The rapidly dividing keratinocytes are pushed up into the prickle cell layer and they look like tiny, spiny projections. They then stop dividing and begin to produce keratin. As they are next pushed into the granular layer, they accumulate a granular substance that is a precursor to keratin. They become clearer and take on a semi-fluid substance, forming a clear, translucent layer immediately under the outer, horny, layer. When they are pushed to the surface they have become flat, flaking cells of dead keratin. These five layers renew themselves every 15 to 30 days.

The dermis is much thicker than the epidermis and contains numerous nerve endings, blood and lymph vessels, sebaceous and sweat glands, hair follicles and tiny muscles. This is the living layer where most problems, including acne, arise, and most metabolic, sensory and other functions of the skin take place. The eccrine sweat glands and the network of tiny blood vessels in the dermis are essential to control body temperature. These produce the rush of heat that a woman experiences during a menopausal hot flush, by suddenly dilating.

The layer of tissue under the dermis contains fat for insulation and energy reserves and the surface which connects the skin to the muscles. This fat also helps convert androgen manufactured by the adrenal glands into oestrogen.

Hair

We usually think of humans as being relatively hairless but in fact we have as many hair follicles as our distant ancestors the gorillas and other apes. Most of ours are the colourless, down-like vellus hairs that cover the entire body except for the soles, palms and skin around the various body openings and nails. The more visible and thicker 'terminal' hairs are found on the scalp, and as eyebrows and eyelashes.

At puberty, vellus hairs on specific parts of the body develop into terminal ones and on men they are on the face, chest, arms and legs.

While women have the follicles, the hairs do not develop, though there may be a few coarse ones, on their upper lips, chins, around the nipples and other parts of the body. These are usually due to heredity, but if they are large in number it may be a sign of hormonal imbalance and disease.

At week 12 a foetus has all of its hair-forming structures. At the bottom of the hair follicle's bulb-like structure is the germinal matrix which produces rapidly dividing cells that are pushed upwards. The further they move from the nourishing blood vessels of the dermis the harder they get by producing more keratin. They change into either the middle cortex with pigment cells or the outer corticle made of scaly, dead cells. Some hairs have a medulla in their centre made of softer keratin like the skin's outer layer. The shaft is made of dead cells and the root of living cells.

Hair growth goes in cycles. In the growing phase the cells in the germinal matrix divide rapidly, and as the new cells are pushed upwards through the hair shaft, the visible hair becomes longer. Generally, the hair on the scalp and face grow the fastest and longest, and more slowly and for less time on the arms, usually for two to four years when the breaking down stage starts. This second phase lasts only a few weeks and cells at the root's base become keratinised and club-shaped, reducing blood supply leading to withering and death of the hair. Phase three is marked by a shedding of the old hair as a new hair bulb forms in the follicle bottom. At any given time a third of the hair is in one of these three phases.

A single scalp hair may survive from two to six years. Cutting the ends of hair does not stimulate new growth. With age, scalp hair thins and after menopause women will notice this, but they do not experience male baldness. Hormones determine what hair is where. Androgens stimulate pubic and body hair in boys; they are also responsible for baldness in men. Reduced oestrogen causes facial hair in women after menopause.

Fingernails and toenails

Nails are also formed early in the foetus, getting their pink coloration from capillaries in the underlying dermis. On the average, nails grow about 0.5mm per week, the middle fingernail growing the fastest, the little fingernail the slowest. Our nails grow faster in the summer than winter.

Fact and fiction

Moisturisers soften and soothe but cannot feed what is, by definition, outer, dead cells. Skin nutrition comes from the blood cells in the dermis. Some substances with a small molecular structure can be absorbed through the skin but the molecules of collagen (said to tackle wrinkles) are just too big.

As we grow older, the skin loses some of its elasticity and moisture. Heredity, climate, tobacco, the sun, hormonal balance and overall health determine how quickly skin ages. If your mother has soft skin, you will too probably. Damp climates with little sun are good for skin whereas dry and sunny climates can make skin leathery and wrinkled. Smokers get wrinkles at an early age, perhaps because smoking lowers oestrogen levels.

Claims that hormone creams, usually containing oestrogen, can restore the skin's youthful glow are false. This glow comes from sebum and too much in adulthood simply means an oily skin. While a facelift is a physical tightening of sagging, excess skin and wrinkles, it is not permanent and the same is true of the effect of collagen injected into the wrinkles.

Moisturisers cannot restore dried, cracked skin. Rehydration is achieved by soaking the skin in water and then applying a barrier cream to prevent evaporation.

Mild soap and water are all that are needed to cleanse the skin. Most soaps are a combination of fats and lye, adjusted for the pH balance, and which soap is a question of personal preference. All will remove dead skin and bacteria which may cause body odour.

Since hair, like skin, is dead, it does not need to be fed. It is naturally strong and durable, so keeping it clean and tangle-free keeps it in condition. Under a microscope you can see a thin film of oil covering a structure of tightly overlapping cuticle cells whose tips point upwards. Split ends are caused by the separation of cell layers and back-combing, blow-drying, chemical dyes; perms lift or swell the overlapping cuticle cells. The shine on hair comes from the even reflection of light off the oil-coated cells. Conditioners which return the cuticle cells to their original position and coat the hair with oil will make it look shiny but they do not feed the hair or restore its natural protein. You also have to make sure that detergents in shampoos are well rinsed out of the hair.

People with skin conditions like psoriasis may require a special shampoo but anti-dandruff formulations have little value unless you do not want to wash your hair very often. Shampoos remove the flaking which occurs on everyone's scalp and the more you have the more you need to shampoo. Beer, eggs, protein and other additives may work for some people but they may lessen the shampoo's cleansing properties.

Pigment cells give hair its colour. Melanin is brown-black and predominates in hair that is dark or ash-hued; phaeomelanin, which is yellow-brown, predominates in hair that is red, auburn or golden-hued; greying is due to a gradual reduction in pigment. When pigmentation stops, hair will have become white. Stress or illness can reduce pigment production and hasten the greying process but it takes many months and does not occur overnight. Natural colour cannot be restored. When hair falls out, perhaps during chemotherapy, it may grow back with a colour, even if it was white before, and it may be different from its original colour.

Nails are not made stronger or more supple by consuming gelatin or other protein products; oils, etc. applied to the nails, cannot 'feed' them. Dry, brittle nails may be caused by ageing, exposure to chemicals or drying agents, including excessive use of nail-polish removers and adhesives. Disease can also cause a variety of nail problems including grooving, changes in shape, brittleness and loosening.

Hormone-related disorders of skin and hair

Few seem to pass through puberty without some acne, perhaps for a few months, though some are bothered by it for life. Primarily a condition of adolescence, you can develop acne as a young adult, and it may come and go till menopause. It is probably more significant psychologically than medically.

Hormones play an unknown role in acne and androgens may be somehow implicated. Hormonal changes tend to cause flare-ups in women who have acne – menstruation, the pill, pregnancy, menopause, even stress can worsen the condition. Heredity also appears to be a factor.

Young people with acne can take comfort that cleanliness, or a lack of cleanliness, has nothing to do with acne – the process starts deep in the dermis. Large amounts of iodine or bromides, may provoke a flare-up. Other practices that have been wrongly associated with causing acne include masturbation and other sexual

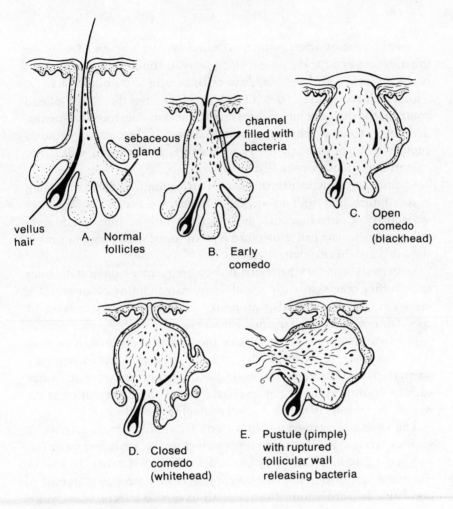

vellus hair

A. Normal follicles

sebaceous gland

B. Early comedo

channel filled with bacteria

C. Open comedo (blackhead)

D. Closed comedo (whitehead)

E. Pustule (pimple) with ruptured follicular wall releasing bacteria

Figure 20. How acne develops

activity, too much or too little sleep and constipation, among many other imaginary causes.

Acne arises in the sebaceous glands that are linked to the hair follicles, in particular in the face and on the upper back. Their sebum, a waxy substance made up of fatty acids, cholesterol and dead cells, carries dead cells to the skin surface, where they can be shed, and also lubricates the skin and hair.

Hormones and bacteria play their roles in the development of acne. The sebaceous glands are particularly sensitive to androgens and their surge during puberty may be why it appears more in boys than girls. Severe acne is often accompanied by the micro-organism

Corynebacterium acnes, which is found in the hair follicle. In the initial stages of acne the pores which serve as the sebum passageways become blocked with sebum, dead cells, keratin and follicle bacteria. This produces a plug, comedo, which blocks the duct. In a closed comedo, the duct opening is blocked at the skin's surface and the underlying comedo is whitish or skin-coloured. If the comedo expands enough to poke through the pore opening, a blackhead will form, coloured by pigment cells, not dirt.

In more severe acne, pressure builds up within the comedo, causing it to rupture and spill its contents under the skin. This leads to inflammation, infection and pus-filled pustules or pimples. Severe, inflammatory acne can cause scarring but this differs between people since it is genetically controlled.

Sometimes acne can be controlled by frequent washing with soap and 'buffing' the skin with a slightly abrasive pad or cleanser. This helps dry the skin and also promotes scaling of the outer layer of cells. Squeezing and picking make it worse.

For treatment, exfoliants inflame the upper layers of skin causing the outer layer to peel off. Benzoyl peroxide in 5 or 10 per cent strengths is very effective. Its action can be reinforced with antibiotics such as erythromycin or tetracycline, but not the latter during pregnancy, as it results in mottled tooth enamel in the baby.

The strongest anti-acne medications are derivatives of vitamin A such as retinoic acid or tretinoin which provoke a marked irritating and peeling action. They may be used with benzoyl peroxide, one in the morning the other in the evening. Another stronger vitamin A derivative is isotretinoin. But these all have side effects, some quite serious and sun exposure can cause them to increase the risk of skin cancer, a growing cause of concern to holiday makers.

Hormone manipulation may help. Women on the pill find acne improves. For some though, the mini-pill may cause a flare-up.

Excessive use of skin products has led to the coining of the phrase, 'acne cosmeticus', brought on among women in middle-age who actually had clear skins in adolescence. Exfoliants and water-based or oil-free cosmetics usually clear this up.

Hirsutism

Men and women have an equal number of hair follicles with the exception of Oriental women who have less. Testosterone is thought to stimulate the conversion of the vellus hairs to the darker and coarser terminal hairs. This type of hairiness is more common in Mediterranean women who are more dark haired and dark skinned than their Northern European counterparts.

For most women hairiness is more of a cosmetic problem than a medical one. Electrolysis will remove hair permanently by destroying the follicles. Depilation and waxing are temporary measures.

Hairiness related to a hormone imbalance requires medical investigation. Warning signs for such a cause include increased hairiness accompanied by signs of masculinisation, loss of periods, sudden and extreme abdominal swelling and fertility problems. Laboratory tests to measure the total circulating testosterone usually find no difference between normal and hirsute women, but those with abnormal hair growth will have almost twice as much free, or active, testosterone which can be readily used by the body.

Disorders that can alter a woman's testosterone balance are many, but rare. The most common involve change in ovarian function. At certain times of their menstrual cycle, some women need to shave their legs and underarms more often. This is natural when testosterone is slightly elevated and oestrogen is low.

Women who stop ovulating will notice a greater increase in hairiness. A typical example might be a woman who starts vigorous exercise training or goes on a crash diet. If her percentage of body fat declines enough for her to stop ovulating, she will notice that she is more hairy than usual.

Overweight women may also develop hairiness because of excessive fat tissue. Menopause often increases facial hair due to the lack of ovulation.

Disorders of the adrenal glands can also cause a rise in testosterone, as can drugs containing androgens, progesterone and hydrocortisone, and drugs such as anti-seizure, anti-hypertensive and anti-psychotic preparations.

Correcting the cause of excessive testosterone will not solve the problem of hairiness. This is because the conversion of a vellus hair into a terminal one is a permanent and irreversible change, as already said. It will remain dark and coarse for life and unless the underlying balance is sorted out, electrolysis will not solve the problem. The active testosterone will simply convert more velli into terminal hairs.

205

Abnormal loss or lack of hair

With age, women experience a certain amount of hair loss or thinning. But conditions such as a high fever can 'shock' all hair into the third of the cycle's phases and cause it to be shed at the same time rather than at different phases for different hairs. Chemotherapy, X-rays, frostbite or burns can have this effect.

Occasionally a child reaches the age of puberty and fails to develop armpit and pubic hair, even though she may develop breasts. This may be a sign of a chromosomal abnormality in which the woman is lacking normal reproductive organs. This is rare but if suspected should be checked immediately, and hormone treatments may correct some of the problems.

Summing up

Most skin or hair problems are cosmetic rather than serious medical disorders. Some hormonal imbalances, however, are reflected in the skin and hair.

GLOSSARY

Abortion: The termination of pregnancy through expulsion of the foetus before it can survive on its own. An abortion may be either induced (also called therapeutic) or spontaneous (also called miscarriage).

Acne: A hormone-related skin disorder characterised by inflammation of the sebaceous glands and hair follicles. Typically it occurs during puberty; comedones, either closed or open, form. The face, neck, and upper part of chest and back are the most common sites.

Acromegaly: A chronic disease in which certain bones enlarge or grow longer after a person is fully grown. Most commonly affects the arms and legs, and the frontal bones of the skull and jaws. The nose and lips also may grow and there is often a thickening of soft tissues of the face. It is caused by too much growth hormone. Treatment is by X-rays to shrink the pituitary; or part of the gland is removed.

Addison's disease: A rare disorder characterised by a lack of adrenal hormones. The adrenal glands are gradually destroyed, usually by an autoimmune disorder or other diseases, such as tuberculosis. Symptoms include fatigue, abdominal pains, lack of appetite, nausea, dizzy spells, a darkening of the skin, and an increased susceptibility to infection or physical stress.

Adipose tissue: Fatty tissue.

Adolescence: The period from the beginning of puberty until maturity.

Adrenal cortex: The outer part of the adrenal or suprarenal gland. The adrenal cortex makes three kinds of vital steroid hormones: corticosteroids, mineralocorticoids and the sex steroids.

Adrenal glands: Endocrine glands just above the kidneys which secrete cortisone and other steroids produced in the outer portion of each gland. The 'stress' hormones, such as adrenaline (epinephrine) and noradrenaline (norepinephrine), are secreted by the inner portion of the gland.

Adrenaline: One of the stress, or catecholamine, hormones produced by the adrenal medulla. Also called epinephrine, it acts to constrict blood vessels, thereby raising blood pressure, and stimulates the heart to beat faster. It also speeds up the release of glucose stored as glycogen in the liver to provide fast extra energy. The body secretes extra adrenaline and other catecholamines in response to danger.

Adrenal medulla: The inner part of the adrenal gland which secretes adrenaline (epinephrine) and noradrenaline (norepinephrine), the 'stress' hormones responsible for the fight-or-flight response in the face of perceived danger.

Adrenocorticotropic hormone (ACTH): Produced by the pituitary gland that controls the adrenal gland's secretion of corticosteroids.

Aldosterone: The major mineralocorticoid produced in the adrenal cortex. Maintains the body's balance of fluids by helping the kidneys conserve sodium and controls levels of potassium in the blood.

Aldosteronism: A condition caused by excessive aldosterone production. The body retains too much salt and excretes potassium, leading to high blood pressure, altered pH of the blood, muscular weakness, muscle contractions, and numbness. Untreated, it can lead to kidney disease and heart failure, also called hyperaldosteronism.

Amenorrhoea: Lack of menstruation.

Amino acids: The nitrogen-containing building blocks of protein used by the body to form muscle and other tissue. Some essential amino acids must come from the diet, while others are manufactured in the body.

Amniocentesis: Test during pregnancy, usually in the second trimester, in which a small amount of the amniotic fluid is withdrawn via a hollow needle and analysed to detect certain genetic, chromosomal or biochemical disorders in the foetus.

Amnion: The thin transparent sac which holds the foetus and the amniotic fluid during pregnancy.

Amniotic fluid: The fluid surrounding the foetus contained in the amniotic sac.

Androgen: Sex hormones secreted by the testes and adrenal glands that produce secondary male characteristics, such as beard growth, muscular development and deepening of the voice. Testosterone and androsterone are the major androgens. Women also produce small amounts of androgen.

Androstendione: An androgen that is secreted by the adrenal glands and which is converted by fat cells into a form of oestrogen.

Androsterone: One of the male sex hormones (androgens). *See also* testosterone and androgen.

Angiotensin: A substance in the blood that causes blood vessels to narrow or constrict, thereby raising blood pressure. Prompts the adrenal glands to secrete more aldosterone. In women, the levels of angiotensin rise following ovulation, which may account for some of the fluid accumulation that occurs during the pre-menstrual phase of the monthly cycle.

Anorexia nervosa: A serious disorder in which a person, commonly adolescent girl or young woman, embarks on extreme self-starvation. Victims have a markedly distorted body image, and a morbid fear of becoming fat. If allowed to progress, it causes a severe loss of weight, amenorrhoea in women, and arrested growth among older children. Anorexia nervosa is believed to be a psychiatric illness, but its true cause is unknown.

Anovulatory cycles: Menstrual cycles in which there is menstrual flow without ovulation. They may occur in young women who have only recently started to menstruate but in whom regular ovulation is not yet established and in older women who are approaching menopause. Other causes include hormonal imbalances. Also called anovular menstruation.

Anterior pituitary (adenohypophysis): The front (anterior) lobe of the pituitary gland, which is at the base of the brain. It secretes hormones that control growth, the thyroid, gonads, adrenal cortex and other endocrine glands. Hormones from the hypothalamus gland control the anterior pituitary.

Arrhythmia: An irregularity in the heartbeat pattern.

Basal metabolic rate (BMR): The amount of energy or calories required to perform basic bodily functions like breathing, circulation, maintenance of body temperature, digestion, metabolism and so forth.

Beta cells: Specialised cells within the islets of Langerhans in the pancreas whose major function is production of insulin.

Biopsy: The microscopic examination of a small sample of tissue. A biopsy is usually used to determine if a growth is cancerous.

Bradycardia: A slow heart rate, usually less than 60 beats per minute. Mild bradycardia may not cause problems, but if the heart rate is very slow, circulation is reduced, leading to dizziness, fainting and, in extreme instances, a collapse of circulation.

Braxton-Hicks contractions: Painless contractions of the uterus before the actual onset of labour.

Breakthrough bleeding: Vaginal bleeding between menstrual periods. This is a common side effect of low-dose or progesterone-only birth control pills.

Bromocriptine: A drug that suppresses production of prolactin. It can also be given to women with galactorrhoea, or inappropriate breast-milk production. It is generally given to women who fail to ovulate because of prolactin overproduction. A related drug is also used to treat Parkinson's disease.

Bulimia: A disorder marked by insatiable appetite and uncontrolled continuous eating. This is followed by periods of depression and self-denial, and in some cases, forced vomiting and laxative abuse to avoid weight gain. Bulimia is thought to be a psychiatric illness, but its cause is unknown. The most common victims are young women, often college students or professionals.

Caesarean section: Surgical delivery of the foetus by means of an incision through the abdominal wall and into the uterus. It is done when it appears that a vaginal birth will be dangerous for mother or baby.

Calcitonin: A hormone released by the thyroid gland to control blood levels of calcium.

Calcium: This is a silver-white mineral essential to building and maintaining bones and teeth. It is also instrumental in blood clotting, proper function of muscles, nerves, the heart, the activation of certain enzymes, and maintaining the permeability of membranes.

Calorie: A unit of energy. Measured by the amount of energy or heat required to raise the temperature of one gram of water one degree centigrade.

Cancer: A general term referring to the uncontrolled reproduction and growth of cells. There are more than 100 different types of cancers.

Candidiasis: A yeast infection caused by the candida fungus. Many common diseases, such as vaginitis and thrush, are caused by candida infestations. A warm, moist environment will aid the growth of candida. (Also called moniliasis).

Catecholamines: A group of chemicals that work as important nerve transmitters and, among other functions, are instrumental in the body's fight-or-flight response. The main catecholamines made by the body are dopamine, adrenaline (epinephrine), and noradrenaline (norepinephrine).

Coeliac disease: An intestinal disorder characterised by failure to absorb digested food, especially foods containing gluten. Symptoms include diarrhoea, malnutrition, bleeding tendency, and low blood calcium. Treatment consists of avoiding foods that contain gluten.

Cervical (Pap) smear or test (also called Papanicolaou test): The microscopic examination of cells or mucus, shed from organs such as the cervix or bronchi, to detect cancer and pre-cancerous conditions. The technique allows early diagnosis of cancer and has helped lower the death rate from cervical cancer.

Cervix: The neck, or the narrow part of the uterus that extends into the vaginal cavity.

Chlamydia: A family of micro-organisms that live as parasites within the cell, and which have characteristics of both viruses and some bacteria. The most common is *Chlamydia trachomatis* in the membráne lining the eye (conjunctiva) and the lining of the urethra and the cervix. The latter is responsible for one of the most common sexually transmitted diseases and can cause pelvic inflammatory disease and fertility problems in severe cases. *Chlamydia psittaci* infects birds and causes a type of pneumonia in humans.

Cholesterol: A crystalline fat-like substance that is instrumental in forming cell membranes in all animals. It is particularly abundant in the brain, nerves, liver, blood and bile. Cholesterol is made in the liver and is essential to the production of sex hormones, nerve function, and a number of other vital processes. Excessive consumption of dietary cholesterol (found only in animal products, particularly meat, egg yolk, etc) and/or saturated fats (those found in red meat, coconut or palm kernel oils) raises blood cholesterol levels.

Chorionic villus sampling: The removal and examination of cells shed by the foetus in the early stages of pregnancy in order to determine genetic and other chromosomal disorders. This test is still experimental.

Chromosome: A microscopic rod-shaped body that develops from the nuclear material of a cell. Chromosomes contain the genes that determine hereditary characteristics.

Clomiphene citrate: A non-steroidal drug used to stimulate ovulation in women whose pituitary and ovaries are capable of normal functioning. Women who become pregnant while taking this drug have an increased chance of multiple births.

212

Collagen: A protein consisting of bundles of tiny fibres which form connective tissue including the white inelastic fibres of the tendons, the ligaments, the bones and cartilage. Collagen also makes up most of the dermis skin layers, and collagen injections are sometimes used to fill in wrinkles, acne scars and other small skin deformities.

Colostrum: A thick, yellowish substance that is secreted from the breast before the onset of true lactation two or three days after delivery. Colostrum is believed to be important in conferring the mother's immunity to certain diseases on the newborn baby.

Comedo, comedones: The greasy plug blocking the opening of the sebaceous gland. Often called a blackhead because of the dark coloration which comes from discoloration of the blocked sebum, not dirt, as is commonly believed. An infected comedo may develop into a pustule or pimple.

Computerised tomography scan (CAT): A painless scanning procedure using multiple X-ray images and computer processing to map internal organs and structures. The technique is used to detect tumours, blood clots, bone displacement and fluid accumulations. It is used mostly to examine the brain, chest, stomach and pelvis.

Conception: The union of the male sperm and female ovum, or egg-fertilisation.

Congenital: A condition that is present at birth.

Conjugated oestrogen: A form of oestrogen, natural or artificial, that can be prescribed to relieve symptoms of menopause, such as hot flushes or vaginal thinning, as well as bone loss; also may be used to treat failure to ovulate. It also provides relief in advanced cancer of the prostate and some kinds of breast cancer.

Conn's syndrome: *See* aldosteronism.

Contraception: Prevention of conception; birth control.

Contraceptive: An agent or device used in preventing conception.

213

Corpus luteum: A small yellow body which develops within a ruptured ovarian follicle. An endocrine structure secreting progesterone, responsible for changes in uterine endometrium in the second half of the menstrual cycle, and important in the development of the placenta.

Corticosteroid: Any one of the hormones made in the outer layer of the adrenal gland (adrenal cortex). Instrumental in a number of important body functions including the proper metabolism of carbohydrates and proteins, and the working of the heart, lungs, muscles, kidneys and other organs. Corticosteroid production increases during stress, especially in anxiety and severe injury. Too much of these hormones in the body is linked with various disorders, such as Cushing's syndrome.

Corticosterone: A hormone produced by the adrenal cortex which is important in metabolism of carbohydrates, potassium and sodium. It is also essential for normal glucose absorption and storage.

Cortisol: The principal corticosteroid. Its many functions include countering the effects of insulin by increasing the liver's output of glucose and increasing conversion of amino acids to glucose, regulating blood pressure by controlling microcirculation, and countering inflammation. It also stops growth in children and adolescents by causing the skeletal bones' growth plates to close. Also called hydrocortisone.

Cretinism: A congenital condition caused by severe lack of thyroid in the baby. Signs of cretinism include dwarfism, mental retardation, puffy facial features, a large tongue, navel hernia, and lack of muscle tone and coordination. Early treatment with thyroid hormone can restore normal body growth, but it may not prevent mental retardation. The use of iodised salt dramatically reduces the incidence of cretinism in a population whose food is lacking in iodine.

Crohn's disease: A chronic bowel disease with swelling and inflammation of the lower part of the small intestine and the colon. Thought to be an autoimmune disorder. Frequently, the diseased parts may be separated by normal sections of bowel. (Also called regional enteritis).

Cushing's syndrome: An overproduction of glucocorticoid hormones often caused by an ACTH-producing tumour, usually of the pituitary gland. People with Cushing's syndrome develop a distinctive moon-shaped face and redistribution of fatty tissue to form a 'buffalo' hump on the upper back, a portly trunk, and thin legs. Symptoms include muscular weakness and wasting, a thinning of the skin, excessive hairiness, weight gain, high blood pressure, increased vulnerability to infection, and in later stages, the development of diabetes. Cushing's syndrome can also be caused by taking large doses of steroid drugs over a prolonged period, as might be the case in severe asthma.

Cyclic adenosine monophosphate (cyclic AMP): A chemical compound important to the action of many peptide hormones and the transmission of nerve impulses.

Cyst: A closed sac or pouch that contains fluid, semi-fluid, or solid material. Many women develop fluid-filled breast cysts. Cysts also may result from obstructed ducts or from parasitic infection.

Cystic fibrosis: An inherited disorder of the glands that secrete through ducts (exocrine glands), causing the release of a thick mucus that can block or damage the pancreas, lungs, and sweat glands. The sweat is excessively salty and bitter to the taste – an important clue in proper diagnosis. The disease is usually diagnosed in infancy or early childhood. It is eventually fatal, but with improved treatments of recent years, a growing number of cystic fibrosis children are living into adulthood, and some are surviving into their 30s.

Cystosarcoma phyllodes: A rare breast tumour which is usually benign, but sometimes malignant. The tumours tend to grow very rapidly and may occupy the entire breast.

Danazol: A drug that suppresses the action of the pituitary gland through androgen-like action.

Deoxyribonucleic acid (DNA): A nucleic acid present in the chromosomes of the nuclei of cells that is considered the chemical basis of heredity and the carrier of genetic information.

215

Diabetes insipidus: An uncommon disease caused by inadequate secretion of vasopressin, a hormone that helps the body retain water. It is marked by excessive thirst and overproduction of urine and is more common in the young.

Diabetes mellitus: A common disorder caused by the failure of the beta cells in the pancreas to produce adequate insulin, a hormone essential for proper carbohydrate metabolism and a number of other important body functions. It is characterised by high blood sugar (hyperglycaemia) and sugar into the urine (glycosuria). Early symptoms include excessive thirst, unexplained weight loss, mood swings, and a general feeling of being unwell.

Diencephalon: The portion of the brain that includes the thalamus, metathalamus, epithalamus and hypothalamus. It is the seat of many basic drives or instincts essential to survival, such as hunger, thirst, sleep, procreation and the instinct to fight for survival.

Diethylstilbestrol (DES): A synthetic oestrogen hormone once given to pregnant women to prevent miscarriages. Its use is believed to have resulted in a higher risk of a rare form of vaginal cancer and other reproductive abnormalities, including difficulty in achieving or main-taining a pregnancy among daughters born to womem who took it. DES is also used to prevent conception if given promptly after unprotected intercourse (the 'morning after' pill). DES alters the uterine lining and thereby prevents implantation of a fertilised egg should conception take place. It is also used in the treatment of certain cancers.

Dilation and curettage (D&C): A procedure in which the opening to the uterus (cervix) is widened and the lining (endometrium) of the uterus is scraped with a curet. A D&C is done to diagnose diseases of the uterus, remove polyps and other small growths, or to correct heavy vaginal bleeding. It also may be used as an abortion technique, or to remove remnants of pregnancy left behind in an incomplete spontaneous abortion, or miscarriage.

Diuretic: Popularly called water pills. Any drug or other substance that promotes increased fluid removal from the body via increased urine production. Diuretics are commonly used to treat high blood

216

pressure, congestive heart failure, oedema, and other disorders with excessive water retention.

Down's syndrome: A congenital condition marked by mental retardation and physical deformities caused by a chromosomal abnormality called trisomy 21. The incidence of Down's syndrome increases among babies born to women over 35 years of age. The disorder was formerly called Mongolism because of the characteristic shape of the eyes and face.

Dysfunctional uterine bleeding: The term refers to uterine or vaginal bleeding that occurs in the absence of ovulation. Sometimes the bleeding may resemble normal menstruation; more often, however, it is irregular and may be heavier than in normal menstruation. Causes include tumours, both benign fibroids or cancer, and hormonal imbalances in which ovulation does not take place. It also occurs in adolescent girls or women approaching menopause, the times of a woman's life in which ovulation may be irregular or absent.

Dysmenorrhoea: Painful or difficult menstruation; menstrual cramps. In about 10 per cent of women, dysmenorrhoea is severe enough to inferfere with normal activities, and may even be incapacitating. In most women, a specific organic abnormality cannot be found, in which case it is called primary dysmenorrhoea. Excessive prostaglandin activity is now assumed to cause the pain, and taking antiprostaglandin drugs (ibuprofen and other anti-inflammatory drugs commonly used to treat arthritis) will relieve the cramps for most women. Secondary dysmenorrhoea is menstrual pain that is caused by specific pelvic abnormalities, such as endometriosis, an abnormal tissue growth of endometrial tissue outside the uterus, long-term pelvic infection, chronic pelvic congestion or fibroid tumours.

Eclampsia: A serious complex of problems seen only in pregnancy which includes high blood pressure, swelling or oedema, kidney damage, protein loss, and a tendency toward seizures. Toxaemia of pregnancy can develop as a consequence of the high blood pressure.

Ectopic pregnancy: Implantation of the fertilised ovum outside of the uterus, usually in a fallopian tube. If undetected in its early stages, an ectopic pregnancy may cause a tubal rupture and serious abdominal bleeding.

Embryo: The early stage of foetal development during which the various organ systems are formed. In humans it occurs between the second and eighth weeks following conception.

Endocrine system: The body's ductless glands and other structures that secrete hormones into the blood stream, affecting virtually every organ system and bodily function. Endocrine glands include the thyroid and the parathyroid, the pituitary, the pancreas, the adrenal glands, and the gonads. A number of other organs, such as the kidneys, small intestine, lungs and heart, also produce hormones and have endocrine functions.

Endometriosis: A common disorder in which some of the endometrial cells that normally line the uterus escape into the pelvic cavity and form clusters of endometrial tissue. These clusters may become attached to the uterus, ovaries, tubes, colon and other abdominal structures. In rare instances, they may migrate to the lungs or other internal organs. These cells respond to hormonal stimulus during each menstrual cycle and grow and become engorged with blood, as does the normal endometrium. The tissue bleeds and forms scars which can cause pain and fertility problems.

Endometrium: The lining of the uterus in which the fertilised ovum is implanted and which is shed during menstruation if conception has not taken place.

Episiotomy: An incision made in the final stages of childbirth from the vagina downward toward the rectum to prevent tearing of the skin and help shorten the second stage of labour.

Erythropoietin: A hormone that controls the bone marrow's production of red cells. Erythropoietin production rises following a serious bleeding episode, which lowers the number of red blood cells. The hormone is also increased when a person goes to a high altitude and needs more red blood cells to get enough oxygen from the thinner air.

Exocrine glands: These glands release secretions through a duct to the target organ or tissue. Examples of exocrine glands include the sweat glands of the skin or the saliva glands. The kidney, digestive tract and breasts all contain exocrine glands.

Fallopian tubes: The two tubes or ducts in the female reproductive system that extend from each side of the uterus and end near the ovaries. After ovulation, the egg enters one of the fallopian tubes and travels through it to the uterus. (Also called oviducts).

Fascia: Layer or sheet of connective tissue that separate muscles and various organs or other structures of the body. It also surrounds many muscles and helps hold them together.

Fat necrosis: The death of fat cells. The dead cells may eventually become calcified, with fibrous tissue growing around them forming a hard, irregular lump.

Fertilisation: Union of male sperm and female ovum to form a zygote from which the embryo, and eventually the foetus develops. The process of conception.

Fibroadenomas: A relatively common benign breast condition that manifests itself as a lump – usually round, firm, and painless. Typically, a fibroadenoma will move freely when examined with the fingers. Although fribroadenomas are benign, it is not always possible to tell one from a cancer by physical examination alone. Therefore a needle or surgical biopsy may be done to rule out a malignancy.

Foetal alcohol syndrome: A series of birth defects caused by heavy alcohol consumption, especially during the early part of pregnancy. The defects include small head size, facial deformities, mental retardation, heart defects, poor coordination, crossed eyes.

Foetus: In humans, the child in utero from the third month to birth. Prior to that time it is called an embryo.

Fibrocystic disease: A condition in which cysts, normally fluid-filled sacs, develop thick fibrous tissue, forming benign tumours.

Fibroid tumour: Uterine tumours made up of smooth muscle cells, which are most common after the age of 30 or 35. Most are small and slow-growing, and they very rarely develop into cancer. Large, fast-growing fibroids, or tumours that interfere with fertility, bladder function, or that cause excessive menstrual bleeding may require surgery, either removal of the tumours or, if indicated, a hysterectomy.

Fibrosis: A gradual replacement of glandular tissue by inert fibrous tissue. Commonly occurs in the breast, but is not associated with breast cancer.

Fluoride, fluorine: A mineral that helps to form the bones and teeth. In small amounts, such as in fluoridated water, it helps to prevent tooth decay.

Follicles, ovarian: The egg-forming cells in the ovaries.

Follicle-stimulating hormone (FSH): A hormone secreted from the anterior lobe of the pituitary that prompts the ovaries to ripen an egg each month and is also instrumental in making sperm in the male. Also called menotropins.

Gastrin: A gastrointestinal hormone that simulates secretion of gastric acids in the stomach. Eating stimulates its release.

Gene: The basic unit of heredity. Each ultramicroscopic gene occupies a specific place on a chromosome, and is, under certain circumstances, capable of giving rise to a new characteristic, a process called mutation.

Gestation: Period of foetal development in the womb from conception to birth.

Gestational diabetes: High blood sugar that occurs during pregnancy, then disappears as soon as the baby is born. It is a result of a genetic predisposition to diabetes and the stress of pregnancy. Because of the high levels of glucose in the mother's blood, the foetus produces extra insulin, which acts as a growth hormone. Many of these babies are over-sized at birth, often weighing 4kg (9lb) or more. After birth, the baby may be unable to stabilise its own blood glucose levels, and suffer life-threatening drops in blood sugar. A major cause of stillbirths.

Gland: Any organ that produces and secretes a chemical substance used by another part of the body. Ductless, or endocrine, glands secete into the bloodstream. Examples are the thyroid and the pancreas. Exocrine glands are located near their target organs, and have ducts that permit secretion directly to a particular location. Examples are the sweat and the salivary glands.

Glucagon: A hormone secreted by the alpha cells of the pancreas. It stimulates the liver's release and conversion of glycogen into glucose, thereby raising blood sugar and supplying needed energy.

Glucocorticoid: Any of the steroid hormones that promote the conversion of protein to glucose and glycogen. Cortisone is a major example of a glucocorticoid. When used as drugs, glucocorticoids treat inflammation and temper the body's immune response.

Glucose: Blood sugar. The most common monosaccharide (simple sugar) and the main source of energy for humans. It is stored as glycogen in the liver and can be quickly converted back into glucose.

Glycogen: The major carbohydrate stored in animal cells. It is made from glucose and stored chiefly in the liver and, to some extent, in muscles. Glycogen is changed to glucose and released into circulation as needed by the body for energy. *See also* Glucose.

Glycosuria: Abnormal levels of glucose in the urine. Common causes include diabetes and kidney disease.

Goitre: An overgrown thyroid gland, usually seen as a swelling in the neck. Treatment may involve giving anti-thyroid drugs or radio-iodine, surgery, or giving thyroid hormone.

Gonad: Primary sex gland. Ovaries in the female; testes in the male.

Gonadotrophins: Gonad-stimulating hormones which impel the testes or the ovaries to perform their biological functions.

Graves' disease: A disorder characterised by an overactive thyroid and excessive thyroid hormone production. Obvious signs include a goitre and, if untreated, bulging eyes (exopthalmos). Graves' disease, which is five times more common in women than in men, occurs most often between the ages of 20 and 40 and often follows an infection or physical or emotional stress.

Growth hormone (GH): Instrumental in regulating growth. Secreted by the anterior pituitary and its release, which occurs in bursts mostly during sleep, is controlled mainly by the central nervous system. A lack of GH causes dwarfism; an excess results in giantism or acromegaly. Also called somatotropic hormone.

Hashimoto's disease: An autoimmune disorder that damages the thyroid gland, or affects proper thyroid growth. It strikes women more frequently than men.

Hermaphroditism: A rare condition in which a person has both male and female sex organs. It is caused by a chromosomal abnormality.

Herpes simplex: Recurring infection caused by the herpes virus. Type 1 involves blister-like sores usually around the mouth and referred to as 'cold sores' or 'fever blisters'. Type 2 usually affects the mucous membranes of the genitalia and can be spread by sexual contact. In unusual circumstances, either type can cause damage to other parts of the body such as the eyes or brain. Also, the distinctions between type 1 and type 2 herpes is not as clear as once thought. Either virus can cause genital or oral sores.

Hirsutism: Excessive body and facial hair. In women, the hairiness occurs in a masculine pattern, and is particularly noticeable on the face, chest, and lower abdomen. Common causes include heredity, diseases characterised by hormonal imbalance, and as a side affect of medication.

Hormone: A chemical that is produced by the endocrine glands or tissue which, when secreted into body fluids, has a specific effect on other organs. Often referred to as chemical messengers, they influence such diverse activities as growth, sexual development and desire metabolism, muscular development, mental acuity, behaviour and sleep cycles. Hormones are also instrumental in maintaining the proper internal chemical and fluid balance.

Hormone-receptor assay: A test that measures the sensitivity of cancer cells to hormones, commonly used in breast cancer treatment. The test measures the sensitivity of cancer cells to oestrogen, and to a lesser degree, progesterone. The test helps in the treatment of certain breast cancers by hormonal manipulation.

Human chorionic gonadotrophin (hCG): A hormone released by cells in the placenta – the tissue connecting the mother and foetus. After fertilisation, hCG prompts the corpus luteum to continue to secrete oestrogen and progesterone to establish and maintain the pregnancy. Early pregnancy can be detected by measuring a rise in hCG.

Human growth hormone (hGH): A hormone secreted by the pituitary which is the major hormone controlling growth after birth. A failure of the pituitary to produce adequate hGH results in pituitary dwarfism, in which the person has a normal body shape, but is abnormally small.

Human placental lactogen (HPL): A hormone produced in the placenta which stimulates the breast to begin milk production.

Hydrocortisone: A hormone isolated from the cortex of the adrenal gland; also prepared synthetically. Its effects are similar to those of cortisol.

25 Hydroxycholecalciferol: The precursor to the active form of vitamin D, which assumes hormonal function by promoting the absorption of dietary calcium from the intestines and also increases the kidneys' reabsorption of the mineral.

Hyperaldosteronism: An overproduction of aldosterone which causes excessive sodium retention and high blood pressure, as well as a depletion of potassium, which can cause irregular heart beats, muscular weakness and cramps. Also called aldosteronism.

Hypercalcaemia: An excessive amount of calcium in the blood.

Causes include bone cancer and other bone disorders, excessive para-thyroid and thyroid hormones, or overdoses of vitamin D.

Hyperplasia: An overgrowth of tissue due to excessive proliferation of normal cells. Common examples include cervical hyperplasia, which is an overgrowth of cervical tissue.

Hyperthyroidism: Overactivity of the thyroid gland leading to excessive production of thyroid hormone. Symptoms include weight loss, restlessness, signs of Graves' disease, such as abnormal bulging of the eyeballs (exopthalmos), constant hunger, fatigue, rapid and irregular heartbeat, and, sometimes, a goitre.

Hypertrophy: An increase in an organ's size, independent of normal growth, that is caused by an increase in cell size rather than number.

Hypoglycaemia: Abnormally low levels of blood sugar as a result of taking too large a dose of insulin or excessive release of insulin by the pancreas. Symptoms include weakness, headaches, hunger, problems with vision, loss of muscle coordination, anxiety, personality changes, and, if untreated, delirium, coma and death.

Hypocalcaemia: Abnormally low blood calcium.

Hypospadias: A structural defect in which the opening in a man's penis is on the underside, preventing his depositing the sperm deeply enough in the vagina, causing conception problems.

Hypotension: Blood pressure that is too low for normal functioning.

Hypothalamus: The part of the brain just above the pituitary gland. It works in concert with the pituitary to control other endocrine glands and is instrumental in a number of bodily functions.

Hypothermia: Abnormally low body temperature, below 95°F or 35°C, which can lead to a failure of vital organ systems.

Hypothyroidism: Underactive thyroid with inadequate production of thyroid hormone, which results in a slowing down of almost all bodily functions. It is sometimes caused by surgical removal of all or part of the thyroid gland, an overdose of anti-thyroid medicine, or a shrinking of the thyroid gland itself. It can also stem from a pituitary problem, in which that gland secretes an improper amount of thyroid-stimulating hormone. Common symptoms of hypothyroidism include weight gain, sluggishness, dryness of the skin, constipation, increased sensitivity to cold, and a general slowing of body processes.

Hysterectomy: Removal of the uterus.

Insulin: A hormone secreted by the beta cells of the Islets of Langerhans of the pancreas. The hormone is essential for proper metabolism, especially of carbohydrates, and for maintenance of the proper blood sugar level.

Interstitial cell-stimulating hormone (ICSH): An anterior pituitary hormone that stimulates the testes to produce male hormones.

Ischaemia: A marked drop in blood flow to an organ or body part, often marked by pain and inability to function normally. A common example is ischaemic heart disease, in which a portion of heart muscle does not get enough blood – usually because of atherosclerosis in the artery supplying that area – resulting in chest pain and even a heart attack. Prolonged ischaemia can result in tissue death, as is the case in a heart attack.

Islets of Langerhans: A group of cells (alpha, beta and delta) in the pancreas that secrete endocrine hormones. The alpha cells produce glucagon, the beta cells produce insulin, and the delta cells produce somatostatin. Destruction or impairment of function of the Islets of Langerhans may result in diabetes.

Kallmann's syndrome: A disorder in which the pituitary fails to secrete the hormones that stimulate the production and release of gonadotropins. Boys with this disorder may have undescended testicles and lack normal male sex characteristics; girls do not develop breasts or other female characteristics. It also is associated with the loss of the sense of smell.

Ketone bodies, ketones: Highly acidic substances produced in the body as a result of normal fat metabolism in the liver. Ketones provide fuel for muscles. Excessive production of ketones, as may

225

happen in poorly controlled diabetes, leads to their excretion in urine and a potentially dangerous buildup in the blood. Also called acetone bodies.

Ketosis: The buildup of ketones, which are highly acidic substances, in the body. This condition is often associated with poorly-controlled diabetes and can lead to a fatal coma.

Klinefelter's syndrome: The most common of the male gonadal abnormalities. Men have small, hard testes and impaired sperm production. Some fail to develop secondary male characteristics, and instead, develop breasts and have little or no body hair. They also suffer from mental retardation or psychological problems. The underlying defect is the presence of an extra X chromosome.

Lactase: An intestinal enzyme important in the digestion of lactose, or milk sugar.

Lactose: A complex sugar found in milk and milk products. It is converted to glucose and galactose by lactase, a digestive enzyme.

Lactose intolerance: Intolerance to milk caused by a deficiency of the enzyme lactase which is essential to the absorption of lactose from the intestinal tract. Symptoms include abdominal cramps, intestinal gas and discomfort. Not so common among Caucasians, it frequently develops as a person grows older, although it also can be present from birth.

Laurence-Moon-Biedl syndrome: A developmental disorder associated with low levels of gonadotropin hormones and characterised by retinitis pigmentosa, a progressive eye disorder, extra fingers, toes and undeveloped gonads.

Luteinisation: Process of development of the corpus luteum within a ruptured follicle following ovulation.

Luteinising hormone (LH): A hormone secreted by the anterior pituitary that is instrumental in reproductive function. In men, it stimulates the testes to produce testosterone, the male sex hormone which acts with the follicle-stimulating hormone (FSH) in prompting the testes to produce sperm. In females, luteinising hormone, working together with FSH, stimulates the ovary to secrete oestrogen. High levels of oestrogen cause a surge of LH which stimulates the release of an egg from the ovary in ovulation.

Luteinising-hormone-releasing hormone (LHRH or GnRH): A substance secreted by the hypothalamus that controls the release and synthesis of two pituitary hormones – the luteinising hormone and the follicle-stimulating hormone.

McCune-Albright syndrome: A disorder affecting the central nervous system resulting in precocious puberty with cafe-au-lait spots, facial asymmetry or skeletal deformity.

Mastectomy: The surgical removal of breast tissue. Part or all of a breast may be removed, together with muscle and lymph tissue.

Mastitis: Breast inflammation, which occurs most commonly among women who are breastfeeding, but it may also be caused by an obstructed milk duct or a bacterial infection.

Melanin: A black or dark brown pigment that occurs naturally in the hair, skin, iris and choroid membrane of the eye.

Menarche: The onset of menstruation during puberty.

Menopause: The end of a woman's ability to reproduce, marked by a gradual cessation of menstrual periods. Menopause occurs between the ages of 40 and 58, with 51 being the mean age. As a woman approaches menopause, menstrual periods become more irregular, and the flow may be lighter or heavier. Ovulation becomes more erratic and there may be hot flushes, night sweats, mood changes and other symptoms, most of which can be relieved by hormone replacement therapy.

Menstrual cycle: A woman's monthly cycle that begins with menarche and ends with menopause. Each cycle is characterised by hormonal changes that thicken the endometrium, the lining of the uterus, and which prepare the body for pregnancy. If conception does not take place, the endometrium is shed during menstruation and a new cycle begins. The average length of the cycle is 28 days, but this can vary from 20 to 35 days or even more, depending upon the individual woman.

Menstruation: A period of uterine bleeding accompanied by shedding of the endometrium. Averages 4 to 5 days in duration.

Metabolism: The combination of chemical and physical changes in the body essential to convert food to energy and other substances needed to maintain life.

Metastasis: The spread of disease – usually cancer – from one body part to another, usually via the blood or lymph systems.

Metrorrhagia: Irregular and excessive menstrual bleeding.

Mineralocorticoid: A class of steroid hormones secreted by the adrenal cortex that affect sodium and potassium balance. Aldosterone is the primary example.

Mitosis: The process of cell division.

Mittleschmerz: Pain experienced during ovulation which may range from a mild twinge to severe cramping.

Myomectomy: The surgical removal of a fibroid tumour, most often from the uterus.

Myxoedema: A severe form of thyroid deficiency which, if untreated, may lead to coma and death.

Nipple papillomas: Wart-like growths in a milk-duct lining near the breast nipple. They usually produce a bloody discharge, and may be felt as a small lump near the nipple. They occur most often in premenopausal women.

Nipple polyps: Small benign growths that form on the nipple skin. They often resemble tiny mushrooms, with a thin stalk and rounded head. They are not cancerous.

Nisidioblastoma: A growth disorder, present at birth, in which babies tend to be very large, with very large tongues and often an umbilical hernia. The excessive growth is attributed to overproduction of insulin due to a pancreatic tumour. Once the tumour is removed, normal growth is generally achieved.

Nonsteroidal anti-inflammatory drugs (NSAIDs): Used in the treatment of arthritis, these drugs are also effective in preventing or relieving menstrual cramps for up to 90 per cent of women who suffer from dysmenorrhoea. A common example is ibuprofen, which is available in both prescription and non-prescription strengths.

Noradrenaline: A stress hormone, produced by the adrenal medulla, and nerve endings. It increases blood pressure by narrowing the blood vessels.

Oedema: Swelling of body tissue caused by a buildup of fluid.

Oestradiol: The most potent form of natural human oestrogen. It is secreted mostly by the ovarian follicle, and also by the placenta, and perhaps by the adrenal cortex. It is responsible for development of secondary sex characteristics in adolescent girls; it also promotes the growth of the endometrium during the first part of the menstrual cycle.

Oestrogen: One of a group of steroid hormones responsible for the development of female secondary sex traits (such as breast development). Human oestrogen is produced in the ovaries, adrenal glands, testicles and both the foetus and placenta. Oestrogen prepares the wall of the uterus for fertilisation, implantation and nutrition of the early embryo.

Oral contraceptive: An oral steroid drug for birth control. The two major steroids used are progestogen only (the mini pill) and a combination of progestogen and oestrogen.

Orthostatic hypotension: Unusually low blood pressure that occurs when a person stands after sitting or lying down, causing dizziness and light-headedness. In some people, the sudden drop in blood pressure may cause the person to faint. Also called postural hypotension.

Osteomalacia: Softening of the bones due to a lack of mineralisation. The bones become flexible and deformed and often are often seen in people with kidney failure.

Osteoporosis: Bones become thin and porous as a result of calcium loss. Occurs most frequently in post-menopausal women, especially the small-boned of northern European extraction, and those who smoke. It usually can be slowed or prevented by oestrogen replacement therapy and calcium.

Ovaries: The female reproductive glands whose function is to produce the eggs (ova) and the sex hormones estrogen and progesterone.

Ovulation: The periodic ripening and rupture of the mature follicle and the discharge of the ovum, which is then ready for fertilisation by the male sperm.

Oxytocin: A pituitary hormone that stimulates the uterus to contract, thus inducing labour. It also acts on the breasts to stimulate the release of milk.

Pancreas: The gland situated behind the stomach which has both endocrine and exocrine functions. Its secretion of enzymes and pancreatic juices plays an important role in digestion. Specialised clusters of endocrine cells (the Islets of Langerhans) secrete insulin and glucagon, hormones that are essential in the regulation of carbohydrate metabolism and blood sugar levels, and somatostatin, a hormone important in regulating growth.

Parathyroid glands: Small endocrine structures, usually four in number, that lie on the back and sides of each thyroid lobe. Their parathyroid hormone is instrumental in regulating the level of blood calcium.

Parathyroid hormone (PTH): Released by the parathyroid glands to keep a constant level of calcium in the body and its excretion in the urine. Loss of the parathyroid glands results in low blood calcium, leading to muscle spasms, seizures and death if the hormone is not replaced.

Pelvic inflammatory disease (PID): A serious infection of the reproductive organs that can damage a woman's fallopian tubes, uterus and ovaries. Causes include sexually transmitted diseases, especially gonorrhoea and chlamydia. Use of an IUD by a woman with multiple sex partners also increases the risk of pelvic inflammatory disease.

Phaeochromocytoma: A relatively rare benign tumour of the adrenal gland or (less commonly) the bladder, that secretes adrenaline and noradrenaline, two of the major stress hormones. It causes persistent hypertension; other symptoms may include headaches, sweating, high blood sugar, nausea, vomiting and fainting spells. Treatment is by surgical removal or drug therapy to lower the hormone levels.

Pineal body: A small, cone-shaped gland located on the back of the midbrain. It is often listed as an endocrine gland, but no hormones or definite function have been associated with it.

Pituitary dwarfism: A disorder in which the pituitary gland does not secrete growth hormone, producing an abnormally short child. Sexual development may eventually take place if the pituitary produces the necessary gonadotropins. Some growth can usually be achieved by treatment with growth hormone.

Pituitary giantism: A rare disorder with a very rapid growth spurt during childhood and a change in features – an overgrown lower jaw, a thickening of the hands and feet, and an overgrowth of soft tissue. It is usually caused by a tumour that secretes growth hormone.

Pituitary gland: The pea-sized gland located at the base of the brain. It is controlled by the hypothalamus and it, in turn, controls the hormone production of many other endocrine glands.

Placebo: An inert substance that has no medicinal properties, but which may be given for psychological benefit or as part of a clinical research study.

Placenta: The structure that develops on the uterine wall during pregnancy and which links the mother's circulation to that of the developing foetus. Through the placenta, the foetus receives nourishment and oxygen and eliminates waste products. It is expelled from the mother as the afterbirth following delivery of the baby.

Placenta previa: Placenta which is implanted in the lower uterine segment and covers part or all of the cervical opening. If the placenta covers all or most of the cervix, a Caesarean delivery is usually performed to prevent excessive bleeding during labour.

Polycystic ovary syndrome: A disorder with complex hormonal imbalances, resulting in failure to ovulate and infertility. During the monthly cycle, one or more ovarian follicles will swell, but no egg is released. Women with polycystic ovaries also may have abnormal growth of body hair and weight gain. Also called Stein-Leventhal syndrome.

Precocious puberty: Puberty before the age of nine in boys and eight in girls. It has a number of causes, the most common being a tumour affecting the hypothalamus. Others include hormonal imbalances and disorders affecting the central nervous system.

Prednisolone: A potent anti-inflammatory drug derived from a synthetic glucocorticoid hormone. It is used to treat many diseases characterised by inflammation and/or an immune response. Severe asthma is a common example.

Pre-menstrual tension (PMT): A variety of symptoms, both physical and emotional, associated with the menstrual cycle, usually occurring in the week before menstruation.

Pretibial myxoedema: A rare thyroid-related skin condition – usually a part of Grave's disease – in which a raised reddish rash or lumps develop on the front of the legs and top of the feet. The lumps are painless and are usually cleared up with cortisone creams.

Progesterone: A steroid hormone secreted by the corpus luteum, adrenals or placenta. It rises during the second phase of the menstrual cycle and is responsible for preparing the endometrium to support a pregnancy. If conception does not take place, progesterone production drops and the endometrium is shed in the menstrual flow.

Progestin, progestogen: Any of a group of hormones, released by the corpus luteum, placenta or adrenal cortex or similar synthetic substances, which have progesterone-like effects on the uterus. They are now used together with oestrogen in post-menopausal hormone replacement therapy.

Prolactin: Hormone produced by the pituitary gland that is responsible for initiating and sustaining the production of breastmilk. It also has other metabolic functions that are not completely understood.

Prostaglandins: A group of fatty acid derivatives present in many tissues including the prostate gland, menstrual fluid, brain, lungs, kidney, thymus, seminal fluid and pancreas. Extremely active substances affecting the cardiovascular system, smooth muscle and stimulating the uterus to contract, among many other functions. They are also instrumental in carrying out many other hormone-mediated functions.

Pseudohermaphroditism: A condition in which a person has the body traits of both sexes, but has either male testicles or female ovaries (not both).

Puberty: The developmental stage during which secondary sex characteristics appear and reproductive organs become functionally active. In girls, puberty is marked by breast development, the onset of menstruation and ovulation. In boys, it includes growth of the penis and testes, increased muscle mass and deepening of the voice. Both sexes experience rapid growth, changes in body configuration and growth of pubic and axillary hair.

Relaxin: A hormone secreted during pregnancy which acts on the pelvic ligaments during labour, enabling the birth canal to widen so a baby can be born.

Renal erythropoietic factor (REF): A hormone produced by the kidneys that helps control the production of red blood cells in the bone marrow.

Ritodrine: A drug that stops premature contractions.

Secondary sex characteristics: Any of the visible bodily features of sexual maturity that develop as a child enters puberty and matures. In girls they include growth of breasts and increased fatty tissue and the growth of pubic and axillary hair.

Somatomedins: Insulin-like growth factors believed to control the action of the pituitary's growth hormone. Their precise role is not fully understood, but these growth factors are thought to be important in a number of diseases.

Somatostatin: A hormone that controls growth and helps to control the release of certain other hormones. Also called growth-hormone-release-inhibiting hormone.

Somatotropic hormone, somatotropin: *See* Growth hormone.

Soto's syndrome: Also referred to as cerebral giantism, this rare disorder, whose cause is unknown, is present at birth. Children are taller than average at birth and grow rapidly during the first few years of life. Puberty occurs early. Includes a large, elongated head and jaw, large ears, prominent forehead, slanted eyes, below normal intelligence and poor coordination.

Spermatozoa: The mature male sex or germ cell that is formed within the seminiferous tubules of the testes. When it unites with the female ovum, fertilisation takes place.

Stein-Leventhal syndrome: *See* polcystic ovary syndrome.

Steroid hormones: The sex hormones and hormones of the adrenal cortex. These include corticosteroids (e.g. hydrocortisone), the mineralocorticoids (e.g. aldosterone), androgen, oestrogen and progesterone.

Stilbestrol: *See* Diethylstilbestrol.

Tamoxifen: A drug that counters the effects of oestrogen. It is used to treat advanced breast cancer in pre-menopausal women whose tumours are oestrogen-dependent. It also may be given to women with fibrocystic breasts to reduce lumpiness and relieve the swelling and pain.

Testicles, testes: The pair of primary male sex glands enclosed in the scrotum. They produce the male sex hormone, testosterone, and spermatazoa.

Testosterone: The male sex hormone, which induces the secondary sex characteristics.

Thelarche: The beginning of breast development at puberty.

Thymus: A gland that lies behind the breast bone and which is instrumental in immune system function during early life. Its function is not fully understood, but as a child approaches maturity, the gland shrinks and is only a remnant in adults.

Thyroid: A butterfly-shaped gland that lies over the windpipe and just below the larynx. Thyroid hormones are essential to numerous metabolic processes essential for early growth, regulation of the heartbeat, temperature control and other functions.

Thyroid-stimulating hormone (TSH): A substance released by the front lobe of the pituitary gland which controls the release of thyroid hormone. Also called thyrotropin.

Thyrotropin-releasing hormone: A substance of the hypothalamus that stimulates the release of thyroid-stimulating hormone from the pituitary gland. Also called thyrotropin releasing factor (TRF) and TSH releasing factor.

Trophic hormones: These hormones have no direct action of their own; instead, they stimulate other endocrine glands to go into action and secrete their hormones. Gonadotrophins which stimulate the ovaries or testes to release their hormones, are major examples.

Turner's syndrome: A chromosomal disorder in women, characterised by short stature, failure to mature sexually and, depending upon the chromosmal pattern, a variety of birth defects that may include mental retardation.

Uterus: The female organ, commonly called the womb, in which the foetus develops from the time of conception until birth.

Varicocele: A varicose vein in the testes which can block the passage of sperm or promote male infertility by raising the temperature within the scrotum.

Vasomotor instability: Hot flushes caused by changes in hormone levels affecting the temperature-regulating centre of the hypothalamus. They are a common sympton of menopause. They also may occur when taking certain drugs, such as high-dose niacin to lower blood cholesterol.

Vasopressin: A posterior pituitary hormone that controls the muscle tone of blood vessels and acts as an antidiuretic hormone to conserve body fluids.

Von Recklinghausen's disease: A disorder affecting the central nervous system and characterised by development of brownish cafe-au-lait spots, overgrowth of the sheaths encasing the nerves and other fibrous tissue, seizures, visual defects and mental retardation. Puberty may be either premature or delayed.

INDEX